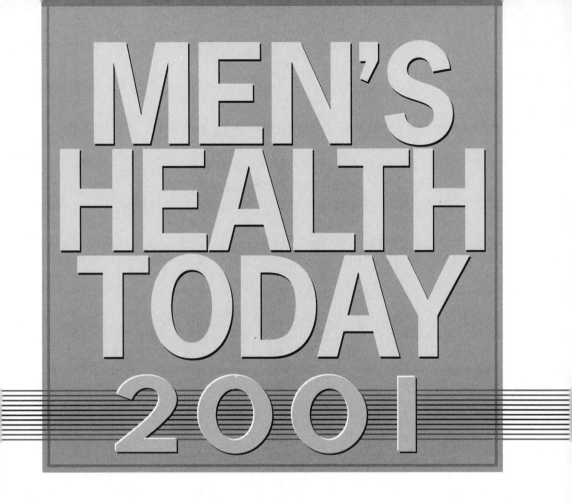

MEN'S HEALTH TODAY 2001

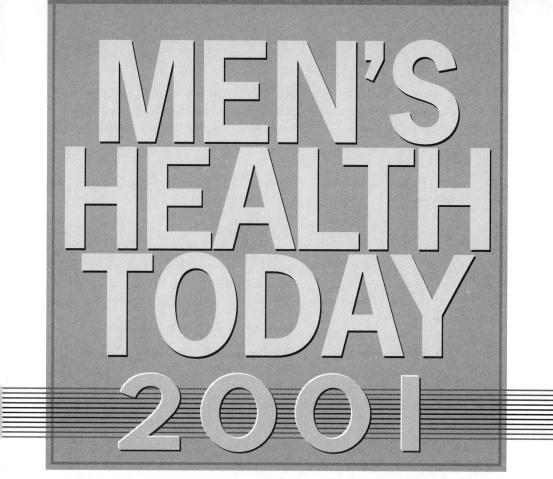

MEN'S HEALTH TODAY 2001

The Best New Thinking and Advice about What Matters Most: Your Body, Your Health, Your Relationships, Your Mind

By the Editors of **Men'sHealth**® Books

RODALE

© 2001 by Rodale Inc.

Illustrations © 1998 by Chris Gall

All rights reserved. No part of this publication may be reproduced or transmitted in any form or by any means, electronic or mechanical, including photocopying, recording, or any other information storage and retrieval system, without the written permission of the publisher.

Men's Health and *Men's Health* Books are registered trademarks of Rodale Inc.

Printed in the United States of America
Rodale Inc. makes every effort to use acid-free ∞, recycled paper ♲

ISBN 1–57954–359–6 hardcover

Distributed to the book trade by St. Martin's Press

2   4   6   8   10   9   7   5   3   1   hardcover

Visit us on the Web at www.menshealthbooks.com, or call us toll-free at (800) 848-4735.

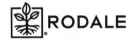

RODALE
WE **INSPIRE** AND **ENABLE** PEOPLE TO IMPROVE
THEIR LIVES AND THE WORLD AROUND THEM

EDITOR, *MEN'S HEALTH* MAGAZINE: David Zinczenko

EDITORS: Amy K. Kovalski, Christian Millman, John D. Reeser

WRITERS: Chris Ballard, Brett Bara, Adam Bean, Ethan Boldt, Kristen Chanley, Rick Chillot, Lucinda Chriss, Warren Christopher, Walter Conway, Amy Donohue, David France, Ron Geraci, Brian Good, Megan Othersen Gorman, Melissa Gotthardt, Jennifer Haigh, Thomas Incledon, Janis Jibrin, Joe Kita, Greg Kohn, Len Kravitz, Ph.D., Richard Laliberte, Michelle Lee, Noah Liberman, Matt Marion, Anna Maxted, Christopher McDougall, Michael Mejia, Christian Millman, Terry Mulgannon, Roberta Naas, Martin Padgett Jr., Larry Platt, Donald Charles Richardson, Lou Schuler, Ted Spiker, Bill Stump, Duane Swierczynski, Joanna K. Trapp, Mariska Van Aalst, Julia VanTine, Zachary Veilleux, Donovan Webster, Debra Wein, Stephanie Williams, Selene Yeager, Tom Zoellner

ART DIRECTOR: Charles Beasley

COVER DESIGNER: Christopher Rhoads

PHOTO EDITOR: James A. Gallucci

PHOTOGRAPHER: Mitch Mandel/Rodale Images

ILLUSTRATOR: Chris Gall

ASSISTANT RESEARCH MANAGER: Sandra Salera Lloyd

PERMISSIONS: Lois Guarino Hazel, Kathryn Piff

RESEARCH EDITOR: Kathryn Piff

COPY EDITOR: Barbara A. Kohl

EDITORIAL PRODUCTION MANAGER: Marilyn Hauptly

LAYOUT DESIGNER: Keith Biery

MANUFACTURING COORDINATORS: Brenda Miller, Jodi Schaffer, Patrick Smith

Rodale Active Living Books

VICE PRESIDENT AND PUBLISHER: Neil Wertheimer

EXECUTIVE EDITOR: Susan Clarey

EDITORIAL DIRECTOR: Michael Ward

MARKETING DIRECTOR: Janine Slaughter

PRODUCT MARKETING MANAGER: Kris Siessmayer

BOOK MANUFACTURING DIRECTOR: Helen Clogston

MANUFACTURING MANAGER: Eileen Bauder

RESEARCH DIRECTOR: Ann Gossy Yermish

COPY MANAGER: Lisa D. Andruscavage

PRODUCTION MANAGER: Robert V. Anderson Jr.

DIGITAL PROCESSING GROUP MANAGERS: Leslie M. Keefe, Thomas P. Aczel

OFFICE MANAGER: Jacqueline Dornblaser

OFFICE STAFF: Susan B. Dorschutz, Julie Kehs Minnix, Tara Schrantz, Catherine E. Strouse

Contents

FITNESS

SEX

EATING

WEIGHT LOSS

Introduction

You Have Been Chosen

At some point in the past, you made a mighty discovery. Maybe it was a decade or two ago. Maybe it was only a couple of years. Could be that it was just this morning. Whenever it was, and regardless of whether the realization crept up on you or hit you all at once, the lesson was the same: You unearthed the remarkable idea that today need not be the same as yesterday.

This, in turn, means that no matter how stagnant you've been up to this particular point in time, you are always free to better yourself—to grow and learn and shake off the sticky cobwebs of lethargy.

And just how do we know you've made this discovery? Simple. You're holding a copy of *Men's Health Today 2001* in your hands. The very act of doing that signifies that you've decided to improve yourself, in all senses of the word. And take it from us, as fellow men, we know—we *know*—how easily you could have left things as they were.

Too many of us choose to start our day washing down a stack of cigarettes with a half pot of coffee. Too many of us choose to fire cheeseburger after cheeseburger into our guts until we're trailing special sauce. And too many men spend more time watching the tube than honing their bodies, more time polishing their cars than their sense of sexuality, more time sharp-ening their ride-on mower blades than their mental steel.

Not you. You chose otherwise. *Men's Health Today 2001* is our way of applauding and encouraging that decision. We jammed it full of the latest and best information you'll need to maintain and even improve your lifestyle.

It all begins with your body. You heard it here first: It's hard to live well if you're dead. Profound, huh? But you get the point. Nothing else matters much if your body can't get you where you want to go. And not only should it get you there, it should rise to any challenge you encounter on the way. So we'll fill you in on how to get the most out of your workouts, how to eat to fine-tune your biological engine, and how to keep your immune system pumped.

That's only the half of it. You'll also find cutting-edge information on how to enjoy that body you're working so hard on. That means information on sex, for starters. For what is manhood if not the ability to linger well within the curves of your partner? Let us show you some new tips on doing just that.

Yet what defines us as men is as much mental as anatomical. The way we approach the world, and succeed in it, depends in large part on our mindset. Look no further for the top new strategies on dealing with stress, earning the respect of your peers, and staving off something no man wants to talk about—depression.

And here's something that *every* man at his peak wants to know how to use to maximum advantage—that elusive commodity known as style. You know immediately when you size up a guy whether or not he has it. The good news is that a sense of style is a learned behavior. Sure, it's partly about the nuts and bolts stuff—clothes and proper grooming. And we'll tell you about that. But it's also about how to present yourself in an assured way. It's definitely *not* about being perfect. If you want proof of that, check out our piece on body flaws that women love.

Some more cool things you'll find inside:

Every guy wants to know how he stacks up against other men. We do it automatically, whether we're playing golf with buddies, checking out a guy's platinum card, or sneaking a peek at someone's leg-press setting. So we created "Benchmarks," a collection of manly averages and oddball facts. You want to know how long it takes an executive to size you up for a job? We have it. The average number of seconds a (sober) 40-year-old can balance on one foot? It's in here. How about the three countries where women are twice as likely as their American counterparts to expect sex during the first week of dating? Go ahead, find your passport. The info you need will be waiting right here when you get back.

In "Vital Reading," we cull the very best advice from a variety of top sources—like the NFL's secrets for injury relief, the world's best weight-loss machine, and even the top foods to take on your commute. And when there's a great new book you should know about, we excerpt a chunk of it in "Best Reads." So you can see why monogamy doesn't have to mean monotony. How to sound smarter than you are when you're in unfamiliar territory. How to keep your prostate plump and happy.

"News Flashes" are exactly that. Your local paper may have ignored or given summary treatment to breaking health news for men, but we don't. This is information from the forefront of the scientific world. Learn why you should sleep in when you want to, how your waist size can determine your risk for colon trouble, and where you should go to dramatically increase your odds of surviving lung cancer.

Those are the most current headlines, but in "Soon to Be News," we pull out our crystal balls to give you a preview of the amazing discoveries hovering in the near future. You may well be able to have yourself vaccinated against ulcers. Or immunized against tooth decay. How'd you like to pop a pill and not worry about getting a woman pregnant? Check it out.

And what kind of health authority would we be if we didn't warn you off the crap that many a huckster would love to sell you? That's what "Fad Alerts" is for. Of course, in cases where the newest tool or pill on the market actually does have some merit, we'll let you know that too.

"New Tools" is a favorite of ours. Did you know there's a baseball glove that measures the speed of your fastball? Or that you can avoid the embarrassment of a doctor's visit with an at-home kit that tells you if you have a sexually transmitted disease? "New Tools" is where we bring you up to date on such nifty, useful items.

We're particularly proud of the fact that guys turn to us for answers to their health questions. They know they can get the straight scoop by sending a letter to the editor or swinging over to our Web site and asking us electronically. In "The Answer Man," we compile the best of these from the last year so you can use these insights to your benefit. You'll find answers to questions like why winter makes you fat, how to wash your wool ball cap without ruining it, and—very impor-

tantly—why dark beer won't give you a hangover.

Rounding out the lineup, we have a great section called "Actions." This goes back to what we were talking about earlier: "Actions" gives you tips you can use to change your lifestyle for the better—right now. You've already demonstrated that you're open to change. We just hope to point you in the right direction.

We enjoyed packing this book to the rafters with great stuff. Use it to help you tweak the beard of time. Because today *doesn't* have to be just like yesterday. And for the man who knows where he's going in life, tomorrow can always be better than today.

Christian Millman
Editor, *Men's Health* Books

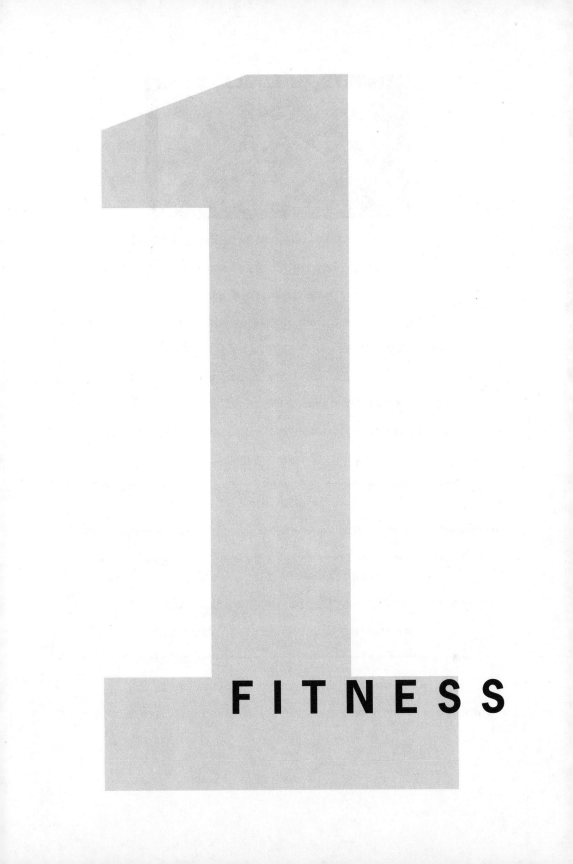

1

FITNESS

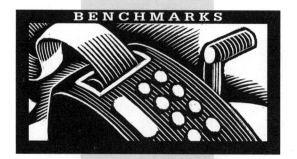

■ Number of new golf courses open for business in 1999: 509

■ Average age of persons who use a personal trainer: 37

■ Their average income: $75,000

■ Percentage of fitness centers offering boxing classes in 1999: 69

■ Percentage of fitness centers offering boxing classes in 1996: 24

■ Top exercise video: Tae-Bo Workout

■ Most utilized equipment in the gym: free weights

■ Percentage of men who are physically active during leisure time: 83

■ Skier to snowboarder ratio: 3:1

■ Number of emergency-room visits in 1997 by elderly Americans injured while snowboarding: 75

■ Estimated number of American men who suffer from compulsive bodybuilding: 669,000

■ Number of acres within National Parks that the American Hiking Society hopes to preserve for recreational use: 60 million

■ Number of steps a day required to maintain a healthy lifestyle: 10,000

■ Average number of daily steps taken: 2,000–3,000

■ The average number of yards a 175-pound man can toss a football: 50

■ The average number of yards for an NFL quarterback: 65

■ The average number of seconds a sober 40-year-old man can balance on one foot: 9

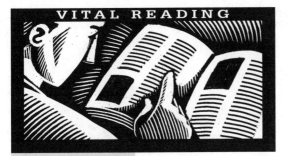

Go Beyond Crunches

Try these two exercises to strengthen your abs like no crunch could.

Most guys think of their abs as one continuous slab of muscle, so they do one continuous set of exercises: crunches. If you really want to etch an impressive midsection, though, it's better to think of your abs as having two distinct sections. Crunches are fine for the top half, but to define what's below the waistband, you need exercises that focus on the hip flexors and the lower half of the rectus abdominis. Add these moves to your workout routine to develop an even tighter, stronger middle.

A couple of caveats: Do the seated jackknife exercise on page 5 at the end of your workout, when your muscles are thoroughly warm, and be sure to stretch your hamstrings between sets. The more limber these muscles are, the harder you'll be able to work your abdominals.

INCLINE LEG RAISE WITH A PULSE-UP

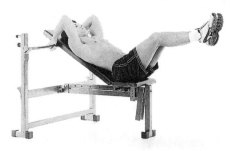

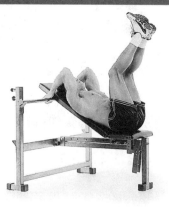

Start by lying on a slant board with your hands gripping the handles behind your head.

Slowly raise your legs until they form a 90-degree angle with your torso.

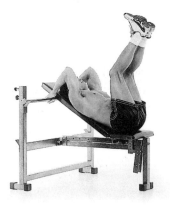

Next, lift your legs toward the ceiling in a controlled pulsing motion; your tailbone should rise an inch or two off the board. Finish by lowering your legs slowly. Do three sets of 10 to 12 repetitions.

SEATED JACKKNIFE

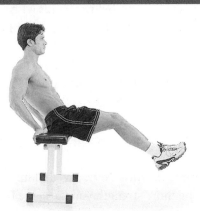
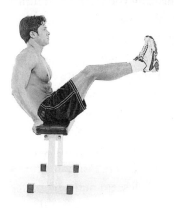

This exercise is guaranteed to rip your lower abs—and you can even do it at home. Sit on the edge of a sturdy chair or bench, holding the seat behind you for support. Extend your legs in front of you and bend your knees slightly.

Simultaneously raise your legs toward your chest and bring your chest toward your knees. Do three sets of as many repetitions as you can manage.

Improve Your Game in 1 Minute Flat

These simple drills will improve your performance in your favorite sport in just 60 seconds.

There's a guy in our gym who's a triathlete, which means he's three times more boring than usual. Sometimes it's better to be really, really good at the one thing you like best.

So we came up with some quick drills and exercises that will help you improve your favorite game. Each will take only 1 minute out of your life. You can do the exercises before, during, or after your main activity without having to spend any more time away from your job, your family, or your pottery classes. And perhaps best of all, they involve no extra laundry.

Running + belly breathing = better endurance. Lie on your back with a book on your stomach. Now inhale. What does the book do? "The book should rise," says Richard L. Brown, Ph.D., a running consultant in Oregon who trains Olympic athletes. "But most of the time, people just expand their chests when they breathe, and the book goes down."

Expanding your chest when you breathe means your diaphragm is rising, squeezing your lungs and limiting their capacity. If your belly expands with each breath, however, your diaphragm is flattening as you inhale, allowing your lungs to inflate fully with oxygen, which will sustain you in the long run.

What to add to your workout: You can practice "belly breathing" anytime, any-place. Just concentrate on expanding your abdomen with each breath. "That develops the neuromuscular patterns that help you breathe correctly when you're running," Dr. Brown says.

Note: It's still very important to suck in your gut, especially when prospective sex partners are present.

Basketball + silly-looking drills = take it to the rack, baby! Weight lifting and basketball seem perfectly paired. After all, the more strength you have, the better you can run and jump and muscle people around under the boards. Right? "Actually, strength doesn't matter in basketball if you can't translate it to movement," says Mike Brungardt, C.S.C.S., conditioning coach for the San Antonio Spurs.

The ideal marriage of strength and movement is plyometrics—explosive jumping drills. These teach your muscles not just to generate power, but to do so as quickly as possible after another movement.

What to add to your workout: After you finish your next game or practice session, try these three drills.

1. Standing long jump: Stand, flex your knees, pull your arms back, and jump as far as you can. Land with your feet together and immediately jump again as soon as you land. Keep going for a series of three or four jumps.
2. Bounding: Travel the length of the court doing a high, bounding skip. Exaggerate every movement so your knees and arms swing as high as possible. Again, take off on the next bound as soon as you land.
3. Triple jump: Start with a standing long jump, but land on just one foot, jump again, land on the other foot, jump again, and finally land on both feet.

These drills should take less than a minute, total, but feel free to build up to multiple sets of each one. Sure, they'll make you look stupid—until you blast past the hecklers and lay in the game winner.

Obligatory words of caution: Don't do these drills until you're warmed up, and avoid them like the clap if you have knee, ankle, or lower-back problems.

Weight lifting + 1 minute of stretching = 20 percent more muscle gain. Maybe more people would stretch if we could guarantee some immediate benefit. Well, we can. "We did a study showing that if you stretch the muscle you're working between sets, your strength gains will be 20 percent greater," says Wayne Westcott, Ph.D., director of the South Shore YMCA near Boston. The subjects in Dr. Westcott's studies were novice lifters, but he says that experienced lifters in a

STANDING LONG JUMP

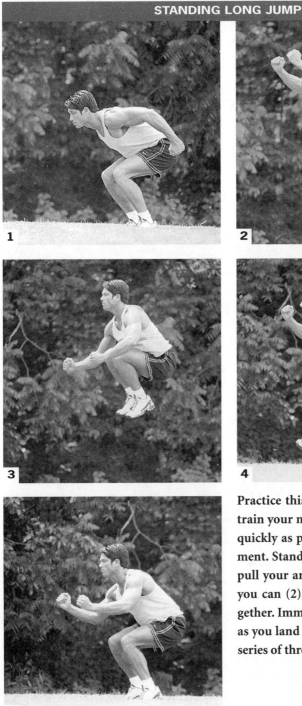

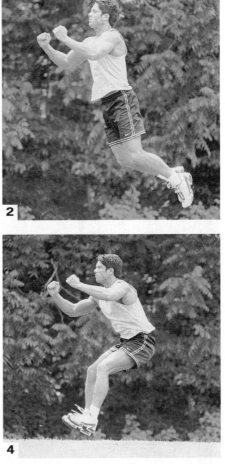

Practice this explosive jumping drill to train your muscles to generate power as quickly as possible after another movement. Stand with your knees flexed and pull your arms back (1). Jump as far as you can (2), landing with your feet together. Immediately jump again as soon as you land (3). Continue jumping for a series of three or four jumps (4, 5).

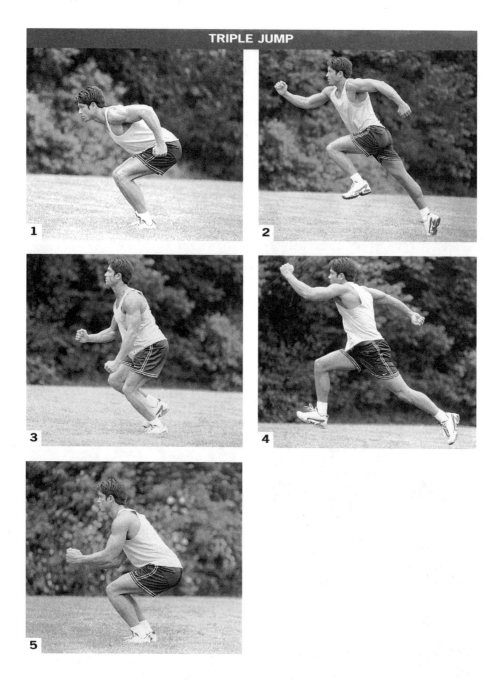

Basketball requires power as well as speed. To improve both, try this triple jump. Begin by standing with your knees flexed (1). Jump as far as you can (2). Land on one foot (3). Immediately jump again, this time landing on the other foot (4). Finally, jump a third time, landing on both feet (5).

New Zealand study discovered the same phenomenon: If they stretched their chest muscles between bench-press sets, they could lift more weight.

What to add to your workout: For 20 to 30 seconds between sets, stretch the muscle you've just worked. You should feel as if the muscle is stretching, but don't push it to the point of discomfort.

Golf + weak-side swinging = longer drives. Golf, like baseball, is a lopsided sport. You're always using one set of muscles to swing from the right or left side, but ignoring the muscles that would help you swing from the opposite side. Normally you'd never exercise this way—you wouldn't do curls with one arm and not the other, or run on just one leg.

That's why the most useful exercise a golfer can do is swing the opposite way, according to Gregory Florez, who trains golfers in Salt Lake City. It helps strengthen and balance your muscles, which might help you clear that water hazard.

What to add to your workout: When you're waiting for your turn at the tee, take a few practice swings from the opposite side. (If you're a right-hander, swing left-handed, in other words.) Since you'll never hit a ball this way, swing easily—start slowly and don't go beyond about 70 percent of your normal swing speed.

You can also do these opposite-side swings for a minute at the driving range, or any other time you find yourself with a club in your hand. (Insert your own adolescent joke here.)

Don't get carried away and exhaust yourself by opposite-side swinging on 18 consecutive tee boxes. A few swings on the first three or four holes should do the trick.

Skating + body-weight squats = more thrust than Ron Jeremy. It stands to reason that more powerful leg muscles translate into stronger skating, whether you want to get up hills when you're inline skating for fitness or beat an opponent to the puck in hockey. "It's like putting a bigger engine in your car. You add power, you add speed," says Mike Boyle, strength consultant to the Boston Bruins.

You don't need to move hundreds of pounds of iron in a gym to build skating-specific leg strength. Boyle says an exercise called the body-weight squat will do the job. A few minutes a week is all it takes to power up your skating.

What to add to your workout: Stand with your feet shoulder-width apart, toes turned a bit outward, knees slightly bent. Focus your eyes straight ahead, and hold your arms however you want—at your sides, straight ahead, around the babysitter, wherever. Stick your butt out, maintain the natural arch in your lower back, and slowly descend until your thighs are parallel to the floor, or almost parallel. Push back up to the starting position and repeat.

Try for a minute's worth of squats every third day, preferably on days when you're not skating. Boyle suggests you build up to 100 total squats a week.

Obligatory words of caution: You should feel the effects in your thigh muscles, not your knee joints. Stop if these squats make your knees hurt.

Swimming + loose ankles = a 10 percent increase in speed. If you've ever used swim flippers, you know what they can do: propel you through the water much faster than you could go without the rubber appendages. But if you develop your ankle flexibility, you can get some of that same propulsive effect, says Mark Schubert, men's swimming coach at the University of Southern California in Los Angeles. At the same time, you reduce the drag that an inflexible foot produces in the water.

A simple 1-minute drill, which you can do anytime and almost anywhere, can improve your kicking and increase your speed by up to 10 percent, according to Schubert.

What to add to your workout: Take your shoes off and sit on the floor. Extend your legs in front of you, your heels resting on the floor. Now point your toes straight out as far as you can, keeping your heels on the floor, and flex your feet back toward your shins. Slowly repeat for a minute, and try to do this drill once a day.

After a couple of weeks, take a deeper plunge: Kneel and sit on your heels, your toes pointing backward. Slowly shift your weight backward until your instep touches the floor and your shin and instep form a straight line.

Your paddle sport + crumpled sports section = invincible elbows. Any dolt can figure out that you need a strong forearm to play tennis well. The problem is how to strengthen it. Play too much tennis and you could end up with tennis elbow. Spend too much time in the gym doing forearm-building exercises and

ANKLE STRETCH

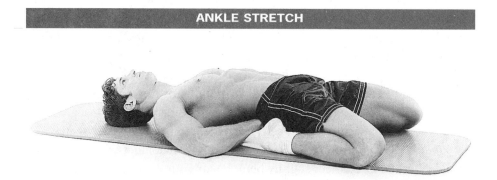

By improving your ankle flexibility, you can use your feet to help propel you through the water as you swim. For an advanced ankle stretch, kneel down and sit on your heels. Your toes should be pointing backward. Then slowly shift your weight backward until your instep touches the floor and your shin and instep form a straight line.

you could suffer other types of overuse injuries in the rat's nest of muscles and tendons that manipulate your fingers and wrists.

The simple act of crumpling a newspaper can build forearm strength with almost no risk of injury, according to Bobby Bernstein, a coach at the USA Tennis Player Development Center in Florida.

What to add to your workout: Lay some sheets of newspaper on a flat surface. Start at one corner of a page and try to crumple it into a tiny ball with your dominant hand. Keep crumpling for 30 seconds, then crumple with your other hand for another 30 seconds, for balance.

At the end of a minute, toss the crumpled balls of newspaper into the air and try to serve them into the wastebasket.

Cycling + one-legged drill = smoother, faster strokes. To the trained eye, an untrained cyclist sticks out like a man at a baby shower. "You see them bobbing up and down and rocking side to side as they ride down the road. People who really know how ride smoothly," says Craig Griffin, the U.S. Olympic cycling coach.

The problem: Inexperienced cyclists hammer down the pedals on every stroke, working their quadriceps over and over without relief. Experienced cyclists pull up on each pedal, using their hamstrings and gluteals, while pushing down with the opposite leg. The way to learn this is to practice pedaling one leg at a time. "It puts the lazy part of your stroke to work," says Griffin. One-legged drills will lead to a smoother, more efficient ride, helping you go farther and faster, and will build more balance between major leg muscles, which will mean fewer overuse injuries over time.

What to add to your workout: To do this drill, you'll need toe clips or a lock-in pedal system. Head out to a lonesome highway (the lonesomer the better; you don't want to worry about avoiding cars). Warm up by pedaling at an easy pace for 5 to 10 minutes. Then let your left leg go limp and stroke with your right leg for 30 seconds. Pedal with your left for 30 seconds while you give your right a rest. Ride normally for 5 minutes, then repeat the 1-minute drill, and continue alternating for 20 to 30 minutes.

The Best Workout:
Aerobics versus Strength Training

At last, the debate is settled between runners and weight lifters. Now you'll know whether aerobics or weight training is king of the fitness hill.

Everyone knows which type of exercise he prefers—aerobics or strength training. But which is better? Exercise scientists split the difference, saying that everyone should do some of both. But we're not satisfied with that answer. Co-champions? Come on! Ali and Frazier never agreed to share anything! We want a winner. So we sent them into the ring for a 10-round physiological grudge match to see which form of exercise does more for physical well-being.

And you've earned a ringside seat.

For the scoring, we used pro boxing's 1 point must system. That means the winner of a round gets 10 points. If the round ends in a draw, each contestant receives 10. A score of 10 to 8 is a blowout—the poor sap with the 8 got pummeled. Ten to 9 means it was close.

Round 1: Bone Strength

Both forms of exercise help your bones stay healthy and strong, but the increases are site-specific. If you run, your lower-body bones stay strong, but you don't do anything to beef up the bones above the waist. Total-body weight training strengthens all bones.

Cardio Guy: 8
Muscle Man: 10

Round 2: Blood Pressure

Here's where inexperience becomes a factor in this fight. The few studies on the effect of resistance training on blood pressure contradict one another. Aerobics, though, clearly heads off the increase in blood pressure that's common as we grow older.

Cardio Guy: 10
Muscle Man: 8

Round 3: Resting Heart Rate

This is a crucial indicator of fitness. Fewer beats per minute means your heart is stronger, pumping more blood with each contraction. Studies on resistance training swing wildly, from no effect on resting heart rate to an 11 percent reduction; in general, it probably won't do much to slow your heart rate. Aerobic exercise may produce reductions of up to 25 percent.

Cardio Guy: 10
Muscle Man: 9

Round 4: Blood Lipids

Here's where the battle swings in favor of cardiovascular exercise. Only really strenuous weight-lifting programs (tough exercises, heavy weights, lots of sets and repetitions) seem to lower total cholesterol and triglycerides and increase HDL cholesterol (the good stuff). But aerobic exercise does all these heart-saving things at any intensity. Even for the guy with the blue headband and matching wrist wraps.

Cardio Guy: 10
Muscle Man: 8

Round 5: Glucose Metabolism

When a body can't process insulin and blood glucose properly—usually due to obesity—blood sugar goes up and diabetes can result. Both weight lifting and aerobics have been shown to improve insulin sensitivity and reduce overall insulin levels. But the nod definitely has to go to aerobic exercise because it uses more calories and increases the clearance of glucose from the blood.

Cardio Guy: 10
Muscle Man: 8

Round 6: Cardiorespiratory Fitness

A knockdown! The skinny challenger is starting to pile up points. Of course aerobic exercise increases aerobic fitness. Weight lifting, with rests of a minute or 2 between sets, doesn't (except for circuit weight training, when performed with very little rest between exercises). Improvements in cardiorespiratory endurance have been linked to increased longevity, so there's every chance that Cardio Guy will outlast his opponent.

Cardio Guy: 10
Muscle Man: 8

Round 7: Resting Metabolic Rate

The muscle mass you add through strength training increases the rate at which you burn calories throughout the day. That means less body fat. For aerobic exercise, the evidence is less clear. Some studies have shown that aerobic exercise boosts metabolism, particularly among elite distance athletes; other studies haven't.

Cardio Guy: 8
Muscle Man: 10

Round 8: Strength

Young, old, healthy, frail—all can see dramatic increases in strength from resistance training. Aerobics? The only strong thing about runners is the smell coming from the gym bag.

Cardio Guy: 8
Muscle Man: 10

Round 9: Functional Capabilities

Which type of exercise helps your body maintain its abilities as it ages? Both. And both, when combined, can improve lower-back health. Going into our final round, aerobic exercise is up by three points. It'll take a knockout for strength training to claim the crown.

Cardio Guy: 10
Muscle Man: 10

Round 10: Longevity

It all comes down to this: Who's more likely to go the distance? A recent study of 18,000 men 45 or older found that the aerobically fittest men outlived the least aerobically fit by almost 9 years. Guys who were only moderately fit had a 6-year edge. So if all you do is lift weights, chances are that Cardio Guy is going to outlive you. Worse, he'll be around to marry your widow and spend your life-insurance payoff.

But do we have a knockout? Nope, because no one knows if there's a direct link between resistance training and longevity. It needs more study. Muscle Man has taken a pounding in this round, but he's still standing as the bell sounds.

Cardio Guy: 10
Muscle Man: 8

The Winner?

Little surprise: Cardio Guy remains champion. But Muscle Man put up a respectable fight, and in a few years, when we've learned more about the health benefits of muscle building, he may even be able to claim the title. If you want the longest, healthiest, most active life possible, do both types of exercise. Meanwhile, if you prefer cardiovascular exercise to weight training, you're allowed a small, superior smirk. Don't get too cocky, though. You may be on track to live longer than Muscle Man, but he can still snap you like a twig. And when was the last time a woman admired the size of your heart muscle?

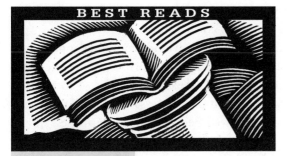

BEST READS

Why the Fitness Bandwagon Has Passed By So Many

Admit it. You've been tempted by one of the myriad muscle supplement, fitness club, and space-age workout machine advertisements out there. You've wanted to shell out the big bucks to down powdered bone meal and unpronounceable amino acids. You've believed in the hype and the promises that you'll be buff within a month for three easy payments of $99.95. Heck, we all have. But here's the truth— for the most part, it's hucksterism at its highest. In this excerpt from The Fitness Instinct *(Rodale), author Peg Jordan shows how the fitness industry has managed to convince people that they no longer know what's best for their own bodies. And, best of all, she assures us that when it comes to movement, we can still be our own bosses.*

It's time to compare the promise to the reality.

For 25 years, the fitness cartel has spent millions of dollars convincing us that the pursuit of hard bodies is the key to happiness. This relentless message has persuaded a few to become full-time fanatics, while the vast majority of us have fallen by the wayside, watching as the fitness bandwagon rolls by. Perhaps you are one of that majority.

Don't feel guilty. It's not your fault if you don't exercise. It's not your fault if your body doesn't look like Arnold Schwarzenegger's. It's not your fault if the thought of pumping iron and generally breathing hard and breaking a sweat makes you want to hide under your bed.

Blame it on the fitness industry.

Much of the reason that you may hate exercise can be attributed to the way fitness has been sold and packaged. A split in the population has occurred between the 20 percent who have benefited from the fitness industry's message and the 80 percent who have been left behind, frustrated and gaining more weight every year. This 20/80 split continues despite a lot of lip service at many health clubs about just going for good health and forgetting about perfection. No matter what is said by the staffs and personal trainers, the emphasis, messages, and images speak louder than the latest politically correct spin.

Two out of 10 people find that the hard-body, muscle-mania approach at clubs is just their ticket. Still, not even those in this minority reap the full benefits of movement. Even these successfully serious exercisers report—both in scientific studies and in my own research—that their fitness pursuits fail to awaken deep, abiding feelings of self-worth and well-being. Rather, their fitness quests often fuel their obsessions about shortcomings and make them feel worse about themselves, their efforts, and their bodies.

As for the other 80 percent, they fall prey to something that I call the intimidation factor, that dreadful sense of shrinking inward and wanting to disappear that you feel when you enter unsafe territory. More than two-thirds of the people I've interviewed talked about the distress they felt when surrounded by "perfect bodies." Diane, a 28-year-old former gymnast, told me that she felt "awkward and incompetent" around the weight equipment, "as if everyone is staring at me, knowing I'm not using much resistance." An older computer engineer told me that he was so embarrassed about his out-of-shape body that he left the gym within a few minutes, without finishing his routine. "The trainers and regulars already have their little clique going. They can't help but hang around and laugh together. I knew that I was the source of their amusement, so I got the heck out. You won't find me exercising around perfect bodies ever again."

Whether or not that perfection was real or imagined is another story. I honestly believe that there is no "perfect body." None of the people I talked to—not even those who had what almost any of us would call perfect bodies—considered themselves to be without imperfections. Even cover models groaned about their skinny calves or their puny wrists or their low-set ears, as if the Earth's rotation depended on their having a different appearance. Why? The pursuit of perfection has been drummed into us with a million images, launching a million obsessions.

Starting at a very early age, girls and boys tend to adopt dieting habits and anxieties about body image based on seductive ads and images designed to sell the perfect body. For years, we all watched Kellogg's Special K commercials in which a slinky torso, the headless woman of a million ads, glided around in a swimsuit. In 1998, however, Kellogg's decided to challenge the stereotypes that have fueled people's insecurities about their bodies. The cereal-maker began creating ads that debunk the ideal body image, announcing that "perfection is about accepting yourself the way you are," says Karen Kafer, the firm's director of communications. A more recent ad features a worried-looking, naked baby girl with a caption balloon: "Do I look fat?"

Self-esteem is largely determined by how people feel about their looks. I didn't want to believe this, and I hoped that self-esteem was determined more by one's education, social support, family ties, and similar high-minded standards. Then I reviewed more than 300 research studies and psychological surveys that convinced me otherwise. At the same time, as a television journalist, I was regularly coached by media consultants who showed me the focus group statistics about what people remember.

When people listen to a speaker, the visual content accounts for 70 percent of what they recall. They pay attention to only about 10 percent of the words. That's why, when Hillary and Bill Clinton went on prime-time TV during the 1992 campaign to talk about surmounting marriage difficulties, all people could talk about the next day was Hillary's hairdo. We're just a little strange that way. Disconcerting as this was, I saw how the fitness industry could easily prey upon this natural tendency to focus on the image and, in turn, let the image affect our feelings of self-worth.

What Is Fitness, Anyway?

Let's be clear about this. Fitness isn't anything real or tangible. You can't go out and buy some "fitness." Nor can you store it, save it for a rainy day, or share it. Some people think that they never have enough of it, although others would look at them and believe that fitness is the main thing they have going for them. Fitness is a concept, a word, an image in the mind, shaped by decades of advances in exercise science along with corporate-sponsored images and publicly broadcast messages. Fitness as a cultural phenomenon is controlled by a cartel that includes several industries, among them beauty, fashion, sports, sporting goods, and media. What is *real* is your life.

It's easy to lose sight of that when fitness is packaged and sold in the image of a mean-looking tigress wearing a very revealing leotard to show off a bosom that defies nature—not to mention gravity—on someone with such obviously low body fat. Just in case the message is too subtle for you, the tigress is usually posed in profile, with her spine dramatically arched and her butt thrust out. This pose has launched many million-dollar aerobics video careers and sold millions of dollars worth of health club memberships, fitness equipment, and clothing. For men, the image of a muscle-bound he-man pumping iron can have the same effect.

These unrealistic and unattainable images can turn you into a mere spectator in life. When you can shake off the spectator trance, however, and return to your own life, you get to explore what fitness can mean specifically for you. In other words, what matters to you physically is your ability to perform all of the activities on a typical day. Now, if your typical day involves a lot of back arching and butt thrusting, perhaps the fitness cartel can help you. If not, it's time to help yourself.

If you had to outrun your food, chasing rabbits and guinea pigs, as do the people of a native tribe in northern Mexico, fitness would imply the ability to sprint like a cheetah every other day. If you earned your daily keep by diving for sponges, you would be fit only if you could hold your breath for 3 minutes. Keeping up a level of fitness that exceeds your present daily activity requires an artificial overlay of exercise. By artificial, I mean any physical effort that is not part of your normal movement repertoire.

We go through our days performing about four or five different movements: stretching, lifting, reaching, walking, and holding. These moves help us to be functionally fit to accomplish what we want. They exercise the entire neuromuscular unit, from brain to limbs and back again. Think of it as a loop of fired-up electrons, a lightning stream of neurons and twitchy muscles, communicating and cooperating. As wellness expert Neil Sol, Ph.D., explains, "Functional fitness is all about strengthening the loop." If that's the case, artificial exercise ignores the loop.

Isolating one muscle with a slow set of carefully tracked biceps curls is, in a sense, an artificial exercise. Rarely in life do you have to use one muscle to do something. The act of reaching for a heavy dictionary and lifting it across a table involves numerous muscles in your shoulders, chest, and arms—more muscles and tendons than you can imagine. Some work as primary movers, others as secondary assistants, and still others as stabilizers. An entire concert of cooperative teamwork takes place.

Time spent performing isolated movements and artificial exercise is part of the cult of body image and perfection obsession. The more hours you invest in this cult, the more you invest in the world of image over substance, looks over function. How did this happen? It happened because fitness became mystified.

The Mystification of Fitness

Making it harder than it is—that's how any profession robs you of your own intuitive know-how. The legal profession invented its own legalese. The medical profession created an aura of "knowing better" about life-and-death issues. Even mortgage institutions know how to make a homeowner's agreement so convoluted that you willingly pay all sorts of fees just to free yourself from the excruciating explanation of details.

The fitness profession is no different. Health and fitness have become mystified, abstracted, and intellectualized. We now must rely on scientists and experts, instead of our own common sense, to figure out how to be fit. I've been asked by countless people, "What should I do if I don't like going to a gym or working with weights?"—as if simple movements such as walking or dancing were somehow beyond their normal experience. They ask, "What kind of exercise should I do if I've got the flu?"—as if they have lost their bodily cues to lie down, rest, and recover. I grow more dismayed every day when I read letters to the editor asking, "Is walking really a good way to exercise?"—as if the simple act and its blood-pumping benefits elude them. Inquirers ask about intensity, "How do I know if I'm working too hard?"—as if they can't tell anymore when their muscles are tired or they are out of breath.

Of course, people believe that they need these answers in order to exercise properly. If you've listened to the countless messages dumped on your doorstep by the fitness industry, you've probably believed it, too—until now. You shouldn't feel like a dope for relying on these fitness "experts" for answers that your body already knows. You've been brainwashed—and now it's time to undo the damage.

Many people have lost touch with their own bodies' yearnings to stretch, move, or walk. Ever since the new breed of experts largely requisitioned fitness training and physical advice, I have discovered in more than 400 interviews how a reasonable person's own self-generating capacity for initiating movement is polluted with embarrassment and insecurity.

The fitness industry has simply made health and fitness information difficult to understand. Mystification takes fitness out of the practical and into the scientific realm, requiring high levels of mastery. Exercise science mastery became the exclusive domain of specialists who had achieved advanced levels of education and experience: sports medicine physicians, exercise physiologists, cardiac nurse specialists, certified technicians—professionals who must interpret the scientific data and write your exercise prescription. This orientation was borrowed from the development of cardiac rehabilitation programs, which blossomed in the 1980s due to the record number of coronary bypass operations.

Government public health officials, together with the American Heart Association (AHA) and cardiac researchers, started identifying the risk factors linked to heart disease. In a scramble to control or lower those risk factors, entire protocols were developed to help people change their behavior. As new findings developed, we altered the programs, but for decades, they stayed fairly consistent in recommending the following strategies.

• Limit dietary fat to no more than 30 percent of total calories.
• Lower cholesterol below 200 milligrams and triglycerides under 120.
• Refrain from smoking.

- Control blood pressure by keeping the systolic reading below 140 and the diastolic number below 90.
- Practice some form of stress management.
- Maintain your ideal weight.
- Perform consistent aerobic exercise.

For years, highly publicized national campaigns shouted that if people would only follow these recommendations, they could beat the odds and lower their risks of heart attacks and strokes. It was only when we had many individuals who were still having heart attacks despite doing everything we recommended that we began to question what other biological, emotional, psychological, and genetic factors might be at work.

When I was a cardiac care nurse, for example, I knew a 40-year-old runner who surpassed every one of those guidelines. He followed a heart-healthy diet, even sprinkling lecithin (a fat emulsifier) on his breakfast cereal. He had the blood pressure of a teenager. He had no family history of heart disease or any other identifiable risk factors. Thus, when he dropped dead from a sudden heart attack, it made me question the value of the numbers game. How do we continue to counsel people to follow set-in-stone guidelines, when every day we see men and women who don't fit the risk factor description yet still succumb to the chief killer of our time?

What the young runner had working against him was the heartbreak of a recent divorce. At that time, grief and loneliness were not part of the scientific profile for heart disease. More recently, however, the case for emotional pain and isolation as risk factors has begun to make its way into the medical literature. It seems that heartbreak is linked to heart disease, and loneliness impacts the immune system.

After working in cardiac care units, I became the cardiac rehabilitation supervisor at a major heart center in Los Angeles; at the same time, I was starting *American Fitness* magazine and writing videos and texts for fitness instructors. It seemed like a perfect segue, since cardiac rehabilitation principles were emulated in the fitness field. Every lifestyle lesson taught to the at-risk population was now being preached to everyone else—now ominously referred to as the "apparently healthy" population. The word *apparently* changed the entire timbre of the fitness movement, allowing nonmedical fitness personnel, armed with the oft-quoted quasi-statistic that "1 in 4 Americans is at risk for heart attack or stroke," to cast a suspicious eye on the average man or woman. (The actual rate is 1 in 1,000, but "at risk" can encompass any number of factors, including stress or physical inactivity.) This misleading statement was latched on to by the health club owners as an advertising ploy, while their staffs scrambled for CPR certification.

The Land of Walking Time Bombs

Clients were seen as "walking time bombs," reported one fitness center employee. "We were scared that they would drop dead of heart attacks during their warmups." Club enrollments included medical disclaimers as well as the usual lawsuit waivers; many clubs followed through with extensive client self-reports outlining medical histories and cardiac risk profiles.

In all fairness, some clients really were at risk for cardiac trouble. For example, I was called as an expert witness to testify against a health club that failed to ask the appropriate questions of a 28-year-old, overweight African-American man who had high blood pressure. After complaining to the staff that he didn't feel well, he was encouraged to take another few runs around the track before going to the steam room. There, he collapsed from a major heart attack and was finally rushed to an emergency room. His rocky hospitalization left him a cardiac cripple, on disability for life.

In their depositions, the club owners talked about the "out-of-shape, unfit characters" and "lazy, unmotivated lard-butts" who "didn't have the proper drive to get fit." I was appalled by their insensitive and self-righteous attitudes, but I knew that the tide had turned against them as far as negligence litigation was concerned. The health club chain settled out of court for an undisclosed sum.

I think about this man now and wonder what could have saved him from a life of baby-sitting his black-and-blue heart. Just how far did he get from knowing what was physically good for him and what wasn't? When he was goaded into taking those treacherous jogs around the track, all the while feeling a crushing pain in his left shoulder and nausea rising in his throat, didn't he stop and think, "This isn't such a good idea; my body can't take this right now"?

I had a chance to ask these questions. This former IBM junior manager is now in his late thirties, still on disability, divorced, and struggling with day-to-day physical exertion. He talked about the tremendous amount of intimidation he felt from the moment he entered the health club. "Everyone was really buff, really in shape. I told them that I had read in their ad in the paper that they had 'personal counselors' who could tailor-make a program for me. I knew I was out of shape. I hadn't done anything since high school, and I knew I had high blood pressure, but they didn't ask any questions. They just told me to go and stand with a group of ladies in leotards and somebody would show us the ropes. I asked them again about the personalized part, but they said that everybody got the same thing in the beginning." So much for individual counseling and tailored training.

He also told me that he reported his discomfort and nausea over and over but was told, "Look, that's just nerves. You're probably looking for an excuse to quit—everybody does in the beginning. Just push through it."

What bothers me most about this response is not the lack of exercise knowledge that obviously produced it but rather the mean-spirited discounting of an individual's genuine fears. I believe unconscionable reactions such as this reflect an arrogance and steel-edged superiority that are fostered by the strength-training and body-shaping cults of the fitness movement. Their script goes like this: "I know what's better for you than you do . . . so just pay up and shut up."

"Is It Okay to Bend Over?"

Some personal trainers consider themselves the priests of the fitness religion, serving as intermediaries between the handed-down commandments of body expertise (to which they alone have access) and you. As a whole, the profession has done a lot of good, but I've interviewed far too many health-club members to not make this critique. Often, the trainers have the last word not only about your protocol and progress but also about what constitutes peak performance for you. In interview after interview, I heard women and men complain that they are "so out of shape" that they need personal trainers to harass them into exercise regimens they hate but believe they should do anyway.

At this point, the fitness cartel has usurped basic body knowledge to the extent that the average person I interviewed believes that she can no longer trust her sensory awareness. "The advice keeps changing every year. I've lost my instinct to know what's good for me," complained Shelly, a mother of two who has been a chronic dieter and sometime gym-goer for more than 15 years. She talked about how she tried to follow exercise classes that promised weight loss but steadily gained 15 pounds a year for quite a while. One year's advice was that fat burning is accomplished through low-intensity, long-duration exercise. Another year's advice was that it is accomplished through overall calorie burn, no matter what the intensity.

People write to health and fitness columnists in newspapers nationwide with questions such as: "What do I do to lose weight?" "How long should I walk?" "Should I jump rope?" "Will dumbbells hurt my back?" As unbelievable as it may seem, I got a flurry of questions regarding the simple act of bending over to tie one's shoes. This quandary was prompted after a leading fitness organization banned "prolonged unsupported forward flexion."

Often, I've been asked to ghost-write question-and-answer columns for celebrities such as Arnold Schwarzenegger and many others. "Supply people with brief and helpful answers to all their questions," was the innocent-sounding proposal. I've done these columns for years in national publications, and the questions seem to grow more and more out of touch. A growing dependency develops whenever I supply people with answers to questions that are best asked of themselves. There is only one response to all of these questions that has integrity: Return the question in an empowering way and help people develop awareness about their own body responses.

That's what I hope to do for you—help you answer your own fitness questions. For instance, here's a sampling of common questions to which you already know the answers.

"What do I do to lose weight?" Ask yourself, "What has worked for me in the past?"

"How long should I walk?" Ask yourself, "How long do I feel comfortable walking?"

"Should I jump rope?" Ask yourself, "How do I feel when I try it?"

"Will dumbbells hurt my back?" Ask yourself, "Does my back hurt now? What aggravates it?"

Reflective questioning helps to establish that you—yes, you—are best-suited to determine how your body feels with movement. Anything short of that fosters dependency and robs you of basic self-knowledge about your body.

There are many well-intentioned professionals in the fitness industry who recognize that the old paradigm isn't working and who are asking for a new approach. I'm on the road quite a bit, delivering speeches, workshops, and keynote presentations to people in the health, wellness, and fitness fields. I'm often asked what I recommend for health and fitness promoters, and I tell them that it starts with the basics: Learn to listen and ask questions first. Just as doctors and pharmacists are learning to drop their arrogance and stubbornness and finally listen to patients, it's important for fitness promoters—who are, in essence, part of an offshoot of the medical profession—to follow suit. I tell them to start any counseling session not with their own agendas and well-rehearsed prescriptions in mind but with a sincere attempt to understand the client's life and goals.

Second, I tell health-care providers that they have to finally understand that the population has split into two groups: the 20 percent who are disciplined in their fitness routines, and the 80 percent who are turned off by it all. I tell them that if health and fitness professionals really want to make a difference, they have to listen to the stories of the 80 percent. It was only by listening closely to those tales that I learned to set aside my own arrogance and judgments as a health professional. I also had to come to terms with the ways that I had helped create and colluded with an industry that reinforced messages and images that were, on second look, at cross-purposes to the happiness and goals of 8 out of 10 people.

In fact, much of the fitness message that I and others were spreading was antagonistic. By dropping what I thought I knew and listening deeply, I started my own journey of self-healing and transformation as well.

Four years of interviewing brought me to my knees professionally, and I knew that I couldn't go on doing what I had been doing. The interviews revealed an unbridgeable gap between the oft-hailed "health habits" that people are supposed to follow and what they are actually able to accomplish each day; between the motivational techniques that we encourage people to employ and the irritating discontent and unhappiness that these techniques leave in their wake. With interview after interview and story after story, I learned and awakened and publicly asked for forgiveness. Further, I also saw what truly does work for those who are able to break away from the fitness cartel's grasp and learn once again to listen to—and trust—their own bodies.

Are You Worth the Effort?

In almost every interview that I conducted, it came down to the same thing. As people started to roll out their long, sad lists of excuses for why they didn't exercise or eat right, they often ended with a shrug of the shoulders, declaring, "It's not worth the effort." Upon further questioning, that statement started to unfold into "*I'm* not worth the effort." Similarly, another discounting phrase, "I didn't try hard enough," often turned into "I'm not good enough." For some it was, "I don't have what it takes." Countless women repeated a similar version: "I don't know what's wrong with me—I just can't stick to the diet and exercise routine they taught me."

What do we have here? An epidemic of low self-esteem? A contagion of self-deprecating remarks permeates the fitness attitude of the average person. I asked many leading health promotion experts what could contribute to this malaise. Nationally renowned professionals such as Pat Lyons, R.N., a leading educator at Kaiser Permanente Health System in California; Steve Ramirez, head of the Fresno County health services in California; and Michael O'Donnell, Ph.D., editor of the *American Journal of Health Promotion*, all agree: The experts have been proselytizing people with the same message for more than 20 years and watching them fail at consistent change. This sets up a cycle of blame and repeat failure that sends people into downward spirals of gaining more weight and becoming more sedentary. One wellness physician at the Veteran Administration's Hospital in Los Angeles described this cycle in this way.

> *It's gotten so that I don't tell anybody what to do anymore—and that's a huge shift for a doctor, believe me. Instead of assigning this ridiculously artificial routine on a Health Rider or some other piece of equip-*

ment that they hate and that is going to be thrown in the garage in a week, I just listen to them about how they conduct their days—where they work, what they like to do when they come home. I'm beginning to think that it all comes down to self-esteem. If they start to feel good about themselves, I can assist that process by showing some interest in them as people instead of seeing them as people who need to alter their entire lifestyles. And that's another thing: Alter for whom? For them, or for me, so I feel better about my medical practice? They've got to make the change from within, and I'm convinced that it actually starts with self-esteem.

The High-Priced Ripoff

To understand how insane the fitness movement has become, consider the case of Gayle, the single mother of a six-year-old boy, who works two jobs just to make ends meet. She has always carried 10 more pounds than she'd like, and late one night, she succumbed to the propaganda of an infomercial selling a $150 walking program. By the time we talked, the question she began to ask herself was, "Do I really need a $150 program, complete with audiocassettes, training heart zones, walking exercise zones, motivational tapes, and life-size posters of walking celebrities—*in order to take a walk*?"

Here is her description of the expensive walking program, endorsed by a fitness celebrity, that she purchased from TV.

> *I was disappointed the minute I got it—not so much in the package but in myself for falling for another gimmick. I mean, look at my day: I run around like a chicken with her head cut off all day, in and out of errands, chasing around like crazy. Then, I finally get home from work, change my clothes, throw some dinner in the oven for my son, Joey, and strap on the headphones to listen to my audio walking program. I figure I can take a quick walk around the block at least. It's been a week since I bought this thing; I'd better use it.*
>
> *I don't have time to read the booklet, which looks like it basically says something about three walking speeds: slow, medium, and fast. Hello?! This is unbelievable. What did I pay for this? I don't want to think about it.*
>
> *Anyway, I can't stand it. I want to get going, but the tape is blabbing about all the safety factors and risks of walking—stuff I should know before I get started. I've wasted about 10 minutes on my front porch and haven't moved a step. Maybe I have the wrong tape. I go back in the house to see if there's at least some music I can listen to, and then I want to break down and cry. What am I doing? Did I really need this to go take a walk?*

No, Gayle did not need to go through this aggravation and expense in order to take a walk. Somewhere along the line, though, she came to believe that other people know better about what is good for her, so she transferred authority outside herself and looked to the experts for answers about something as basic as taking a walk. When we arrived at this insight in her interview, she got teary-eyed and shook her head, saying, "I'm really done with that routine."

Then, as if the universe were serving up a synchronous challenge, the phone rang in her home. Gayle talked a few minutes, asked some questions hesitantly, then wrote down an appointment. She hung up the phone and said, "That was the dentist's office. They said that I need another cleaning, even though I just had one a couple of months ago. But they said I needed one anyway, so I've got an appointment for that. I just hate the way they poke at the gum . . ." She stopped talking, maybe because of the look on my face; then she said, with a shocked look, "Oh, my God, I'm doing it again, aren't I?"

The conditioning is tougher to break than most people realize, but you must break this pattern in order to fully tap into your fitness instinct. I am not saying that you should never ask anyone for help. Obviously, when we are at a stage of initial learning or are not quite competent at a skill, depending on expert advice adds to our knowledge base. Usually, however, we already have the answers. We just need to learn to trust our bodies.

How did it all become so complicated? When did the simple act of physical activity—the birthright of every human—become the guilt-ridden drudgery of endless stair-stepping? "Forced exercise has all the appeal of a prison labor camp," said Cheryl, a marketing specialist who has been dieting and exercising her entire life.

Granted, our sedentary lifestyles are major culprits in the way we have distanced ourselves from normal daily physical activity. "But who wants to sit on a stationary cycle at night after sitting at a computer all day and then driving home on the freeway for an hour?" complained a 56-year-old writer and editor. "I feel like my butt can't take another minute parked on that damn bike. My kids talked me into one of those rowers, and I won't sit on that, either."

Avoiding the Lifestyle Overhaul

Even though we give a lot of lip service to healthy choices, what's happened in today's society is an obsession with the *wrong* ways to live. People tend to focus on the negative, on everything they shouldn't do. The fitness industry counts on our obsession with lifestyle vices.

Fitness counselors at the Duke University Diet and Fitness Center in Durham, North Carolina, know that overhauling your lifestyle for the long term can be next to impossible without yearly "tune-ups," so they established a return visit policy for graduates of their lifestyle education program. One woman who said that she has been overweight all her life knows that she must maintain the daily grind or she will fall off the wagon. "I have to exercise for 1½ to 2 hours every single day, without fail, and I must always restrict and watch every morsel that goes into my mouth," she said. As one of the lifestyle counselors at the Pritikin Longevity Center in Santa Monica explains, "It has to be a daily obsession, or they fail. Those who can commit to that moment-by-moment awareness are the ones who succeed."

Fail at what? Succeed at what? Moment-to-moment obsession? Is this any way to live? It is time to completely rethink how we approach healthy eating and exercise as lifetime pursuits. If it is an uncomfortable, deprivation-oriented approach, all we are doing is waiting to reward ourselves with a return to normalcy. "If we can modify our lifestyles in small, bite-size chunks instead of the great overhaul," advises health promoter Molly Mettler, "we don't go crazy after the diet or just sit on the couch after a month of classes at the gym. The real revolution in changing habits must be motivated from within. We're in the midst of a self-care revolution, and we have to realize that once people are educated with enough options, they generally will find something that suits them and that they can modify easily."

Commuter Calisthenics

We all know we should exercise. *But between trying to appease our bosses and spending enough time with our kids and spouses so they still remember who we are, who has time to work out? According to Kenneth Winston Caine, editor of* Lose Your Gut Now! A Man's Plan for Shedding Pounds and Getting in Shape *(Rodale), you may be able to snatch a few minutes of exercise time from an unlikely part of your day—your commute. This excerpt reveals how you can safely get in some exercise time while getting to and from work.*

Commuting is one of life's necessary wastes of time, like waiting in a doctor's office or number-punching your way through a voice-mail maze. There's simply no way to get where you need to be without unenviable and inconvenient delays.

In the world of commuting, that delay is pretty significant. According to government estimates, the average worker traveling by car spends nearly 40 minutes a day commuting. If he takes a bus, he's looking at more than an hour roundtrip; and if he rides the rails, the commute averages more than 2 hours a day.

To those of us trying to make time for exercise, these statistics certainly seem daunting. Until someone invents a *Star Trek*–style transporter, it seems that the chances for turning commuting time into exercise time are slim. This is unfortunate because losing weight always requires commitment, and commitments take time. How can a man commit time and energy to exercise and other healthy lifestyle changes when he's always stuck in traffic?

Training in Transit

It doesn't have to be an either-or scenario. Whether you're commuting by car, bus, or train, there are ways to turn some of those lost morning and evening hours into workout time, says John Amberge, a certified strength and conditioning specialist and former director of corporate programs for the Sports Training Institute in New York City.

"It won't be anything like a good workout in the gym, of course. But if you can steal 5 minutes a day for exercise, that's almost an extra ½ hour of exercise a week," he says. Commuter workouts make great supplements to a man's regular exercise routines.

Take a look at the gaps in your commuting time, says Sandra Lotz Fisher, exercise physiologist and president of New York City's Fitness by Fisher, a fitness and stress-management consulting firm. "When you're waiting for your ride, anytime you're a passenger in a vehicle, when you're at a stoplight, while you're in a traffic jam—these are all times that you can devote to a variety of exercises without endangering yourself or your fellow commuters," she says.

The Freeway to Fitness

For those who commute by car, doing anything more strenuous than fidgeting seems impossible without ending up on the eye-in-the-sky traffic report as the accident that's blocking the left lane.

"Not so," says Fisher, who developed an audiotape for drivers called "Freeway Flex: Stretch and Tone Exercises to Do While You Drive." "You absolutely shouldn't do it at any point where it's going to take your attention off the road," she adds.

That said, if you drive in light to moderate conditions, there's plenty of time during your morning or evening drive that you can convert to exercise time.

"Gridlock can be your friend," says Charles Kuntzleman, Ed.D., professor of kinesiology at the University of Michigan in Ann Arbor and director of Blue Cross and Blue Shield of Michigan Fitness for Youth Program, also at the University of Michigan. Any time that traffic is at a standstill, that's time you can spend doing a few simple exercises—burning calories instead of brain cells.

Here are a few in-car exercises that you can do while waiting in traffic—not while driving—that will help make your morning and evening commutes an integral part of your weight-loss plan.

Shrug your shoulders. This is a very simple exercise that works out the large trapezius muscles in your back and neck. Hold on to the steering wheel at the 9 and 3 o'clock positions. Push back against the seat until your arms are straight, and raise your shoulders up toward your ears. Do 10, 20, or however many you have time for before traffic starts moving, Dr. Kuntzleman says.

Squeeze the wheel. Grabbing the steering wheel in a death grip loosens muscles in your hands and forearms. If you really go after it, it will build hand strength as well. Hold for a count of five, then relax. "Really focus on the release part," Dr. Kuntzleman says. "That stimulates a relaxation response in the body, which will help you be more loose and limber when you get to work."

Vacuum off flab. Similar to crunches, vacuums are abdominal exercises that you can do while sitting up, Dr. Kuntzleman says. Sit up straight in your seat. Suck in your stomach as though you were on a beach and the Swedish Bikini Team were strolling by. Hold for a count of 10, then relax. Vacuums are harder than they sound. Try to do 5 at first, then work up to 10.

Work the "off" leg. Between brake pumping and gas stomping, your right leg gets a pretty good workout in the car. You can work your left leg by doing a simple toning exercise. Tighten it as much as you can for 3 seconds. Feel the tightness in your quadriceps and hamstring. Then release. You can do a similar thing with your ankle and toes. "You won't have nearly the cramps and sore-leg problems a lot of drivers complain about," Fisher says.

Workouts for Drivers

Maybe driving isn't how you get to work: It is your work. If so, here are three exercises, suggested by Marge Rodgers, a physical therapist and former rehabilitation-services coordinator for Genesis Rehabilitation Services in Baltimore, that will loosen you up, tighten your gut, and burn some calories at the same time.

Stretch your hamstrings. The main muscle in the back of your leg, called the hamstring, always tends to be tight, causing knee and back pain. It pays to keep it loose—even if you're sitting behind the wheel of a tractor trailer all day. Before you climb into the cab, stand by the side of your truck, facing the door. Lift your foot up and rest your heel on the step. Your knee should be straight, not bent. Hold for a few seconds, then relax.

Roll with it. Crunches are among the best abdominal exercises, but you can't do them when you're driving. Here's a gut workout that you can do. Slump in the seat, lift your chest, and push your stomach muscles out. Find the place of maximum tension, then hold the stretch for a few seconds. Relax, then do it again. This exercise is surprisingly effective at stretching and strengthening your abs. "These muscles need to be strong to help support your spine," Rogers says.

Bend over backward. "Every time you get out of the cab, step to the side of the truck, put your hands on your hips, and bend backward, keeping your knees straight," says Rodgers. This will help relax all the muscles in your back, which can help prevent tension backaches from getting started.

Power on the Platform

Transportation schedules being what they are—that is to say, inaccurate— you probably find yourself waiting for your ride a few times a week. The time you currently spend reading can be time spent exercising. Here are a few quick work-outs you may want to try. They'll burn just as many calories as the exercise that you'd do in a gym, and you're doing them in your "free" time.

Pace. "If it's a bus stop, walk up to the corner and back to the stop. Try to do 10 laps before the bus arrives. If it's a train station, try to do as many brisk, walking laps around the station as you can before your train pulls in," suggests Amberge.

Do the bus-stop stretch. Every man needs to stretch, and it's especially im-portant for men who are working out. Dr. Kuntzleman recommends using waiting time to get in some quick stretches. See that chainlink fence near the bus stop? Stand facing away from it. Stretch your arms out behind you, hook your hands into the fence at about chest level, and lean forward. This gives a solid stretch to your arms and shoulders.

Work your calves. Another exercise you can do on any city street is a heel raise. Stand on a curb with your heels hanging off the edge. Slowly rise up on your toes, then lower your weight so that your heels are as low as they'll go. This exercise looks simple, but you'll start feeling the burn after doing two or three. It's very effective for strengthening your calves and stretching your toes and an-kles. It may be hard to keep your balance, however, so it's good to do it near a parking meter or signpost.

Hurry to catch the train. If you commute by train or subway, you probably stand right where you think the doors are going to open. "When you think about it, that's really pretty lazy," says Fisher. She recommends waiting a lot farther away. As the train comes to a complete stop, walk briskly toward the front or back of the train, whichever is farther away. You'll get a quick aerobic hit, and you may even get on faster than if you tried to squeeze your way in with the throng.

Working Out En Route

If you take public transportation, there's no reason to stay locked in your seat. "If you're not doing the driving and you're not packed in like sardines, then you have time and space to do some exercise," Fisher says. Here are some ideas to get you started.

Get off early. Probably the easiest way to convert commute time into exercise time is to get off the train or bus one or two stops shy of your destination and walk or run the rest of the way, Dr. Kuntzleman says. "The way traffic is in most cities, you'll probably get there faster on foot." Just remember to wear walking or running shoes—those executive wing tips won't do you any favors out on the streets.

Stand whenever you can. Men who take trains and buses always head for the first free seat. That's fine when you're reading the paper, but you can burn some additional calories just by being a strap-hanger, says Dr. Kuntzleman.

"Unless you have some back problems or a condition that prevents you from standing for long periods of time, you'll get more exercise from simply standing," he says. The swaying of buses and trains causes muscles to fire in your legs, back, torso, and arms. "It's not a lot, but it's better than sitting and doing nothing," Dr. Kuntzleman says.

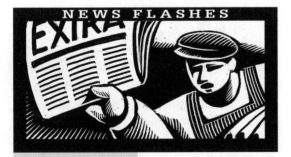

Chromium Picolinate Could Increase Cancer Risk

TUSCALOOSA, Ala.—Bodybuilders have touted them as muscle enhancers, but chromium picolinate supplements may increase your risk of cancer. When researchers at the University of Alabama exposed cell DNA to low levels of chromium picolinate, the DNA became vulnerable to breakage, which may contribute to cell mutations and cancerous changes. "Given the cell changes we saw in the lab, I wouldn't take the stuff," says John Vincent, Ph.D., the study author.

Ibuprofen May Not Be Best Remedy for Sore Muscles

ATHENS, Ohio—According to one study, ibuprofen may not effectively relieve muscle soreness. Eighty subjects exercised to the point of muscle soreness and then received either 400 milligrams of ibuprofen four times a day, 800 milligrams four times a day, a placebo, or no treatment. Over a period of 6 days, none of the subjects reported less pain. Since ibuprofen works by blocking prostaglandins—chemicals that cause inflammation—muscle soreness may stem from some other factor, says John Howell, Ph.D., of Ohio University, the lead researcher. Dr. Howell suggests trying naproxen, which works by a different mechanism.

Time in Gym Not Proportional to Benefits Reaped

PITTSBURGH—Most guys' mantra at the gym is, "Do more to get more." But in a recent study, researchers found differently. Lifters who trained three times a week increased the amount they could curl by 38 percent, while the ones who lifted just once a week increased their biceps strength by 23 percent, according to Philip Bishop, Ed.D., the study author. In other words, the once-a-weekers got half the benefits in a third of the gym sessions. Wish this worked around the office.

Burning Calories May Beat Lung Cancer

BOSTON—Sweating off 3,000 calories a week may help prevent lung cancer. Researchers who examined data collected from 13,905 men over 16 years found that those who burned roughly 3,000 calories or more a week (about 6 to 8 hours of moderate exercise) were 39 percent less likely to develop lung cancer than less active men. They concluded this even after controlling for other factors, such as smoking. "Exercise strengthens the immune system, making it easier to fight off cancer and other diseases," says the study author, I. M. Lee, M.D., of the Harvard School of Public Health.

Lower-Leg Pain May Not Be Shinsplints

ATLANTA—If nothing seems to help your shinsplints, see a doctor. According to research published in the Georgia Tech Sports Medicine Newsletter, a dangerous condition that causes lower-leg pain is often confused with shinsplints. Chronic exertional compartment syndrome (CECS) occurs when leg muscles grow too large for the compartments they're enclosed in. The result is pain during exercise and numbness afterward. "The reduced circulation caused by CECS can lead to muscle death," warns Lyle Micheli, M.D. A simple surgical procedure can have you running within 6 weeks.

Flat Feet Can Increase Risk of Stress Fractures

ROCHESTER, Minn.—Flat-footers already know that their fallen arches can cause joint and lower-back pain. But new research shows that flat feet, or even just lower arches, can increase your risk of exercise-related stress fractures. In a Mayo Clinic study of 449 Navy SEAL trainees, the men with low arches were two times more likely than those with normal arches to develop stress fractures in their feet or legs. "This is the first evidence that suggests that flatter feet can cause stress fractures," says Kenton Kaufman, Ph.D., the lead study author. Ask a podiatrist if prescription arch supports can help pick up where nature left off.

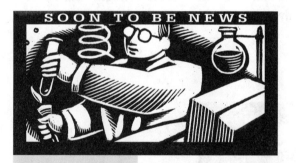

A New Workout Order for Greater Strength?

According to a new study, it could be best to save your stretching for after your workout. When 30 subjects in a Louisiana State and Brigham Young University study stretched vigorously for 20 minutes before a workout, they lost strength during weight training. "Though we're not sure, stretching too hard may relax tendons and make it harder for the muscle to contract at full force," says Arnold Nelson, Ph.D., a kinesiologist and coauthor of the study. This relaxing effect can also cost you speed and coordination. In a Finnish study, 20 men who stretched for an hour before exercising had 85 percent slower reaction times.

Light aerobics, such as running or riding an exercise bike, make a better workout warmup than stretching.

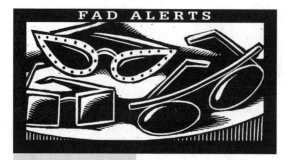

Hoop Harness

If you're right-handed, you tend to do everything with your right hand. This is fine for most activities, but basketball players need both hands to get a strong dribble going. The Hoop Harness ($20) ties up your dominant hand so you'll be forced to work the weak one. We showed it to several Division I basketball coaches, and they liked the principle. "It makes you think about using your off hand," says Mike Brey of the University of Delaware. But there's one big problem. "I'd be afraid to ask anyone to wear it because of the risk of falling without a hand to reach out and soften the blow," he says. For $20 less, use some self-restraint and put your hand behind your back.

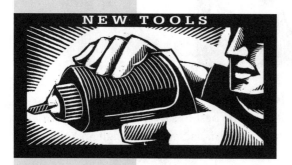

Better Way to Measure the Speed of Your Pitch

Glove Radar

Those computerized baseballs that calculate how fast you throw have one drawback: An unscheduled meeting with a bat can trash them. Glove Radar attaches to the back of your mitt, where it's less likely to be smashed. It senses radar waves bouncing off the ball in the last few feet and calculates the speed from 20 to 120 mph. If you can chuck a ball at 101 mph, you'll beat Nolan Ryan's record. The replaceable lithium battery is good for 5,000 measurements. $80. Call (800) 589-3709, or click on www.gloveradar.com.

Work Out at Home

Peg Board

Remember the peg board in your high-school gym—the one you hung from like an abandoned raincoat? The idea was to climb up or across the board by moving the hand pegs from hole to hole. It was a tough workout that developed your back, biceps, and stomach muscles. Now, if you have a sturdy wall in your basement, you can finally conquer those pegs without having your shorts yanked off by the class bully. BSN Sports in Dallas will ship a 2½-foot-square peg board, with 13 holes and two pegs, for $128. (You'll need four 3½-inch wood bolts to mount it.) Call (800) 527-7510 to order. Just lay a mat on the floor and put on your bike helmet before you climb; your head was a lot harder back in high school.

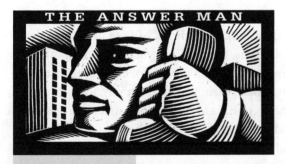

THE ANSWER MAN

Lopsided Lifter

When I do bench presses, my right side seems to be much stronger than my left. How do I correct this?
—L. N., Scottsdale, Ariz.

"It's not unusual for some guys to have one side of their body that's stronger or that has better balance or coordination than the other side," says Hank Drought, C.S.C.S., a personal trainer in Boston. To combat this problem, use dumbbells instead of a barbell when you do your bench presses, and throw in two extra sets of 5 to 12 repetitions to work the weak side only. Because your weak side will already be fatigued, Drought recommends using a lighter weight on the extra sets.

Curious about Curves

I do biceps curls with a straight barbell, but I see lots of guys using a zigzag bar. Which one is better? Is there any benefit to using both?
—K. M., La Jolla, Calif.

The bar that zigs is called an EZ Curl, and it works the same muscles as a regular barbell. "Because of its shape, the EZ Curl bar causes the forearm to rotate slightly, and some lifters say they feel like they're getting a better 'pump,'" says Swapan Mookerjee, Ph.D., of Bloomsburg University in Pennsylvania. "But there is no significant difference in muscle activation between the two types of curls." So there's no advantage to using both bars in your workout, unless you're simply trying to add some variety.

Weekend War Wounds

I go mountain biking or inline skating every weekend, so I get my share of cuts, scrapes, and road burns. What's the best way to prevent scarring?
—M. L., Toms River, N.J.

Whether you develop a scar depends on your skin type, the depth of the cut, and whether it becomes infected, says Brett Coldiron, M.D., a dermatologist in Cincinnati. You can't do much about the first two, but you can prevent infection with some simple first aid. Clean the cut with a mixture of equal parts hydrogen peroxide and water. Dry the skin and apply some petroleum jelly, then cover with a bandage. "The idea that cuts need fresh air to heal is nonsense. Bandages aren't airtight, and studies show that wounds heal faster when they're covered," says Dr. Coldiron. He doesn't recommend using an antibiotic ointment, such as Neosporin, which causes allergic reactions in some people. Another caution: If the cut is so deep that you can see fat below the skin—it looks like lumpy, yellow goo—don't mess around with first aid. Haul your butt to an ER and get some stitches.

Staying off the Disabled List

At least once a year I sprain my ankle as I'm running or playing basketball. Are there any exercises I can do to prevent this?
—N. B., Reading, Pa.

The best way to prevent sprains is to strengthen the muscles on the outside of your legs, says Stephen Pribut, D.P.M., a sports podiatrist in Washington, D.C. The following exercise is done with a Theraband, available at any sporting-goods store. Almost any stretch cord will do, however.

Anchor one end of the cord to a heavy piece of furniture. Sit down, cross your left leg over your right, and attach the other end of the cord to your left foot. Pull your foot and ankle away from the furniture, hold for a moment, and return. Do 14 repetitions, then switch legs. Do one or two sets per leg, three times per week.

While you're running or playing basketball, Dr. Pribut recommends, wear neoprene or elastic braces around both ankles. "This will make you more aware of your ankles, and you'll be better able to tell when the foot is turning in the wrong direction, so you can stop the sprain before it happens," he says.

Jilting the Stilts

Guys at the gym tell me that the best way to build up skinny legs is by doing low repetitions with heavy weights. I've been doing that, but it hasn't been working. Why?
—A. G., Cedar, Iowa

It could be that you need to do more repetitions with less weight. "Lifting heavy weights for low repetitions—five or less—may be effective for maximizing muscle strength, but not necessarily muscle size," says Hank Drought, C.S.C.S., a trainer in Boston.

To make better gains in muscle size, work with weights you can handle for three to five sets of 8 to 15 repetitions with rests of 1 to 2 minutes between sets. Concentrate on multijoint exercises, such as squats or lunges and leg presses. They help you secrete more muscle-building testosterone than moves that isolate muscles, such as leg curls. For a change, you can also ride a bike. Nothing builds muscles like big hills.

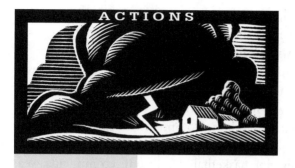

Better sex. A healthier heart. A longer life. Better sex. Toned abs. Did we mention better sex? The benefits of being fit are numerous. The drawbacks of being unfit can be deadly. Any questions? Good, now here's a slew of tips to help get you smartly through your next workout.

1. **If you've been imitating a sloth, start with 30 seconds.** If you've been inactive for longer than you care to remember, start your exercise program with a 2-minute workout, then add 30 seconds a day until you're up to 20 minutes, a half-hour, or hour, wherever you want to be. One minute may seem, well, minute, but it's a start, says Charles Swencionis, Ph.D., director of the clinical health psychology program at Yeshiva University in New York City and coauthor of *The Lazy Person's Guide to Fitness*. And if you add 30 seconds a day, you'll be enjoying the benefits of an impressive 15-minute conditioning routine before a month is up. That's real progress. If you miss exercise for more than 3 days at any point, subtract 30 seconds for each day missed and start over from there.

2. **For a better workout in the bedroom, start jogging.** Sex is not a sport of power; it's one of endurance. So what's the best way to improve your endurance? By improving your cardiovascular fitness with aerobic exercise like jogging, swimming, cycling, or stair-climbing. In a study conducted by James White, Ph.D., professor emeritus at the University of California, San Diego, and author of *The Best Sex of Your Life*, men who performed aerobic exercise reported increases in libido. But more important, they reported having 30 percent more sex and 26 percent more orgasms. "Overwhelmingly, they reported more sexual satisfaction than those who didn't exercise," says Dr. White. Try to keep your aerobic exercise to at least three sessions a week, 30 to 45 minutes at a time.

3. **Put it in reverse to strengthen your obliques.** Reverse trunk twists are great for your oblique abdominals, says John Amberge, a certified strength and conditioning specialist and former director of corporate programs for the Sports Training Institute in New York City. The oblique muscles are the ones you use for push-and-pull activities such as raking leaves or wrestling with the lawn mower.

To do reverse trunk twists, lie on your back on the floor, with your arms straight out to the sides and your palms down. Bend your knees, placing your feet flat on the floor. Now, with legs and feet together, slowly lower your knees to the left until your left thigh touches the floor. Hold for a moment, then raise your legs back to the starting position and switch sides. Do 15 to 20.

4. **Fib about your weight to get a more accurate calorie count.** Most electronic calorie counters on exercise machines are about as precise as a White House spokesman. They can overestimate your calories burned by up to 30 percent, says Michele Olson, Ph.D., an exercise physiologist at Auburn University. But if you're on a machine that lets you input your body weight, you can keep it honest. Key in a weight that's 20 percent lighter than your actual weight. For example, if you weigh 180 pounds, punch 145 pounds into the machine. This will give you a more conservative—but truthful—calorie tally.

5. **Club shoulder pain on the golf course.** Carrying a bag of clubs can turn your shoulders into mush. "What I recommend is that on holes 1, 3, 5, 7, and so on, you carry your golf bag on one shoulder, and that on the even-numbered holes, you carry it on the other side," says Greg Johnson, director of the golf program at Health-South Rehabilitation Corporation in Atlanta and athletic trainer on the Professional Golfers' Association tour. "Most people tend to carry their bag on one shoulder, which not only leaves them sore but also results in their dropping one shoulder—and not playing as well as they could." Or buy a universal strap that allows you to carry your clubs in the middle of your back.

6. **Adjust your feet for a better workout.** Simply changing your foot placement from exercise to exercise can turn a simple leg press into a total leg workout, says Courtney Barroll, a certified personal trainer and medical exercise specialist at Equinox Fitness Club in New York City. Placing your feet as close together as you can without touching, for example, fires the center part of the quadriceps a little more. Placing your feet a little wider apart, about hip distance, and putting pressure on the outer part of the feet emphasize the lateral (outer) part of the quadriceps. Positioning your legs on the outer corners (toes on a slight angle out to take stress off your knees) also works your butt more.

7. **Do a smarter crunch.** Wedge a rolled-up towel under your lower back when you do crunches, advises Michael Mejia, C.S.C.S., a trainer in New York City. This gently curves your back, forcing your abdominal muscles to stretch a little farther at the starting position and contract to a greater degree when you crunch. Also, rest your hands comfortably under your chin as you crunch (placing your right fist inside your left hand). This little trick stops you from jutting your head forward, which can cause a pain in the neck. Adding the towel makes crunches harder, so start with two sets of 10.

8. **Twist your arm for a bigger chest.** If you want to add muscle to your chest, dumbbell bench presses do the job quickly. But one subtle adjustment to the standard move will help you build even more brawn: Try pushing your arms together, not just up. To do this, slowly rotate the weights inward as you push them up, so your elbows are closer together when your arms are fully extended. "This forces your chest muscles to contract more powerfully during the press," explains Wayne Westcott, Ph.D., *Men's Health* fitness advisor. And that means you'll develop more muscle with fewer repetitions.

Grab two dumbbells and lie on a bench with your feet flat on the floor. Hold the dumbbells with your palms facing your lower body, your elbows pointing straight out and bent 90 degrees. As you raise the dumbbells, slowly turn your fists inward so that your knuckles face each other when your arms are fully extended. Contract your chest muscles forcefully for 1 full second, then lower the dumbbells as you rotate your hands back to their starting position. Do two sets of 10 repetitions, and use heavier dumbbells when you can do 12 repetitions easily.

9. **To avoid a pulled muscle, take 10.** Jogging for 10 minutes before you begin your workout can help avoid strains and tears. Jogging gets blood pumping to your legs so they're better able to handle sudden stop-and-start moves. And it's more effective than stretching. Two recent studies showed no difference in injury rates between those who stretched before a workout and those who didn't. Save your stretching until after the workout.

10. **Power up the mountain without getting out of your seat.** Most mountain bikers stand up to generate more power on hills, but your best bet is to stay seated. "When you stand, it takes weight off the back wheel, and you spin out," says Zapata Espinoza, executive editor of *Mountain Bike* magazine. If you gradually downshift before you hit the hill, you'll be able to maintain pedal speed from your seat. Sit back in the saddle and you'll use more of your glutes; sit forward, you'll use more leg. Vary positions to reduce muscle fatigue during a long climb.

11. **Work your back, then your chest.** Before your next set of bench presses, do a set of rows. Your chest contracts more forcefully right after you work your back, so you'll be able to lift more weight and perform more repetitions, says Marc Phillipi, C.S.C.S.

For the set of rows, start with a weight that you can lift no more than 8 to 10 times, but do only four to eight repetitions. Then rest for 1 minute before you begin your set of bench presses.

You can also use the principle of working opposing muscles throughout your workout. Do triceps extensions before biceps curls, for example.

12. **Get roped in.** When you're facing a long upward climb on your morning jog, it's natural to want to look at your feet. (After all, that way you don't have to look at the torturous track ahead.) Next time, though, try this trick instead: Imagine that a rope is attached to the middle of your chest and it's being wound in from a point two stories above the top of the hill in front of you, suggest the editors of *Runner's World* magazine. Lifting your head opens your airways, so it's easier to breathe than when your upper body is hunching forward.

13. **Try this tonic for muscle cramps.** If running gives you nighttime cramps in your calves, drink tonic water before you go to bed. It contains quinine, a plant extract that acts as a muscle relaxant. The FDA banned over-the-counter quinine pills for leg cramps because large doses (above 260 milligrams) can be toxic. But 8 ounces of tonic water contains only 27 milligrams. That's enough to alleviate muscle cramps in some people, says Paul Davidson, M.D., of the University of California. Add lemon to the tonic water or mix it with orange juice to reduce its bitterness.

14. **Take small steps to get the best workout.** It seems logical: If you want to cover more ground fast, take bigger steps. But it doesn't work that way. "The real trick to walking faster and getting the best workout in the shortest time period is to take more steps per minute than you usually walk," says Don Lawrence, who conducts walking clinics for Nike. "Too many people think the key to walking faster is to take a bigger stride, but that is less efficient. A quicker stride can be achieved by counting your steps in 30 seconds. Develop a rhythm to gradually increase the steps per minute."

15. **Get a firmer shake while you're on the phone.** One of the first things our dads taught us was the importance of a firm handshake. So why not work on it while you're on the phone? Many executives have begun keeping small exercise balls, designed for hand strength, on their desks. While you're talking, squeeze the ball with everything you have. Relax for a second, then repeat.

16. **Get in a workout while you're on the clock.** Stuck at work with no time to make it to the gym? Never fear—if you've got a desk, you've got a way to work those triceps. To do a desk pushup, lean forward against the edge of your desk with your hands shoulder-width apart and your palms facing down. Your legs and back should form a straight line, and you should be up on the balls of your feet. Your arms should be slightly bent, elbows unlocked. Press down against the desk. Your elbows should be bent and facing outward. Then press back to the starting position.

17. **If your weight-lifting progress has plateaued, build a pyramid.** This technique can be used to trick your muscles into exerting more effort than they are used to. By lifting heavier and heavier weights in progressive sets, you'll trick the muscle into going beyond the point at which you would ordinarily stop, adding just a little more exertion to each set.

For example, when doing arm curls, start with a pair of dumbbells lighter than you would normally use when doing 10 repetitions. Curl them five times. After a short rest, take the next heaviest set of dumbbells and do five repetitions. Continue up the rack until you reach a weight that is too heavy to curl five times. Then work your way back down through the weights, suggests Dr. Westcott.

18. **Check your old shoes for clues.** When it's time to purchase new athletic shoes—okay, *sneakers*—check out the ways you've eroded your old ones first. If, for example, the back of the heel is worn toward the outside of the foot, you tend to roll along the outer edge when you run (this is known as underpronating). Underpronators have rigid, immobile feet; they should buy shoes that are heavily cushioned and feature soft midsoles and less medial support. These shoes are usually built on a curved form to encourage foot motion.

Overpronators roll their weight to the inside of the foot, so the heel will be more worn toward the inside. It is the more common problem. Overpronators should buy motion-control shoes: rigid, heavy, and durable. Such shoes might include features such as a medial post, a polyurethane midsole, and a carbon rubber outsole. Many are built on a straight shoe form to offer more stability and support.

19. **For a better workout, don't give your muscles a breather.** Most guys alternate dumbbells when they work out. But that way, every time you curl one arm, your other arm has a chance to take a breather. "For the most growth, you should be putting your biceps under continuous tension throughout the whole set," says Michael Mejia, C.S.C.S. Use the following variation instead.

In either a seated or standing position, hold a pair of dumbbells with your palms facing up. With your left arm, curl one dumbbell until your forearm is parallel to the ground; that arm should form a 90-degree angle with your torso. Hold this position. With your right arm, do 6 to 10 curls—each going the full range of motion. Switch arm positions; do two or three sets on each side.

20. **After your workout, try a shower for additional relief.** When you've finished your workout, take a hot shower for 10 minutes, then switch to cool for as long as you can stand it. "The contrast in temperature will increase bloodflow and squeeze out lactic acid, the substance that keeps your muscles from functioning properly later," explains Don Chu, Ph.D., C.S.C.S.

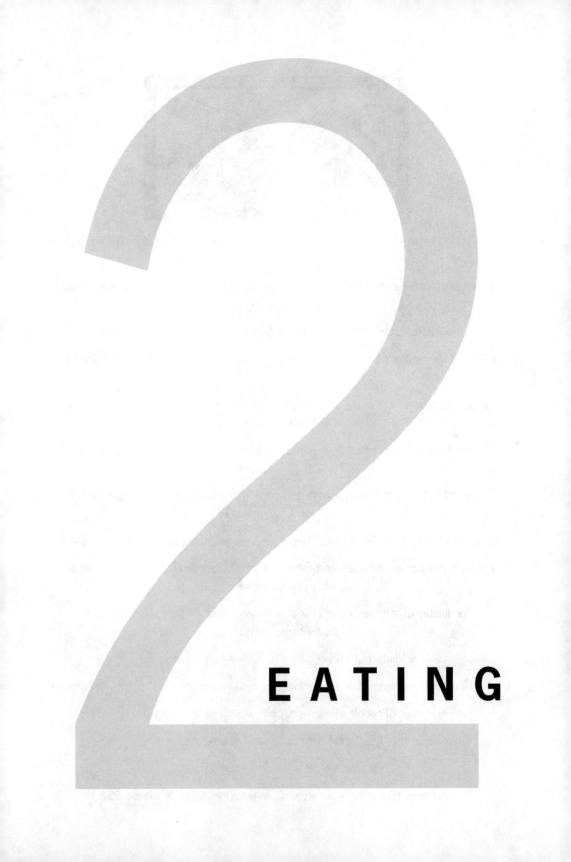

2 EATING

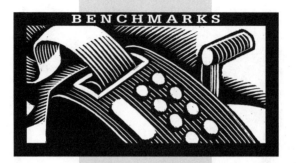

■ Percentage of Americans who've said they would rather take a pill to fulfill nutritional needs instead of eating: 26

■ Percentage of French who've said they would rather take a pill to fulfill nutritional needs instead of eating: 13

■ Billions cut from the five-year federal food stamp budget in 1996: $24

■ Percentage change since 1988 in the amount of seafood eaten worldwide that is farmed rather than caught: 1,146

■ Estimated portion of whale, dolphin, and porpoise meat consumed in Japan last year whose pollution levels were toxic: ½

■ Ratio of annual per capita alcoholic beverage consumption in the United States to that in Russia: 8:3

■ Inches by which today's largest corncobs exceed the length of those grown in 16th-century Mexico: 12

■ Price of a bottle of Czar Nicholas II's champagne salvaged from a ship sunk in 1916: $4,922

■ Rank of broccoli and peaches, respectively, among U.S.-grown produce with the highest residual pesticide levels: 18,1

■ Number of state and county fairs that competed in last year's National Best Spam Recipe Contest : 77

■ Number of cans of Spam consumed every second: 3.1

■ Percentage of Americans who describe "barbecue" as the aroma that best defines America: 39

■ Percentage of people who have thrown away a dish to avoid washing it: 11

■ Percentage less fat in lite cream cheese as compared with full fat: 50

■ Grams of fat in 20 chicken wings: 140

■ Percentage of the world's premium vodka that Americans drink: 55

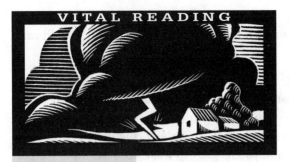

VITAL READING

A Beverage for All Occasions

It's not only solid food that needs your attention.

Guys agonize over the menu—steak or chicken, fries or baked, Caesar or garden—but few of us seriously think about what to drink. "I'll have what he's having," we say. Or we fall back on knee-jerk favorites: a cola, a cold one, a cup of coffee, a cocktail.

But our bodies are 60 percent fluid—108 pounds of a 180-pound man are H_2O—so what we drink is just as important as what we eat. "Staying hydrated and drinking the right thing at the right time can make a difference in how you feel and perform," says Liz Applegate, Ph.D., of the University of California. "Drinking something is the quickest way to nourish, refuel, recover, and reenergize." Consider hitting the bottle in any of these situations.

Situation: Hungry
Remedy: You're on the road, scanning fast-food joints. Head to a 7-Eleven instead, and grab a canned meal replacement, such as Ensure (250 calories, 6 grams of fat) or Boost (240 calories, 4 grams of fat). "They give you much of what you need," says Dr. Applegate. Or have tomato juice. It's thick and satisfying.

Situation: Suffering from indigestion
Remedy: Buy a bottle of peppermint oil and mix a few drops with 2 teaspoons of sugar. Dissolve the mixture in half a glass of water. It should help reduce spasms in your intestinal tract.

Situation: Constipated
Remedy: You need liquid and fiber to spur your cranky colon, so mix a fruit smoothie. Dr. Applegate suggests tossing an orange, a banana, some frozen berries, a handful of All-Bran cereal, some orange juice, and ice into a blender. Pour the concoction into your travel mug and head to work. By the time you turn your PC on, you'll be ready to download.

Situation: Anxious
Remedy: Have a brew, but make it a nonalcoholic beer. The hops will calm you down.

Situation: Unable to sleep
Remedy: Try warm milk, just like Mom used to make. Milk contains L-tryptophan, the same protein that has you fighting for couch space after your Thanksgiving turkey dinner. What to avoid: alcohol. A bottle of cold duck may put you out, but you won't sleep as well and you're likely to wake up—we hope—to pee.

Situation: Overheated
Remedy: Drinking too much water right after exercise encourages your kidneys to excrete it faster. So have a sports drink, such as Gatorade. "Sports drinks contain small amounts of sodium and electrolytes that help direct the water where it's needed most in the body," says Dr. Applegate.

Situation: Finished exercising
Remedy: Recent studies show that both carbohydrates and protein are necessary after a hard workout. So buy a powdered drink mix that has the necessary 4-to-1 ratio of carbohydrates to protein, suggests Dr. Applegate. Or have 16 ounces of orange juice and half a tuna sandwich.

Situation: Sore from working out
Remedy: Here's your excuse to have a dark beer. Heavy brews, such as porters, contain flavonoids—antioxidants that help you recover more quickly from your morning blast-a-thon. But be sure you're properly hydrated before you imbibe. Alcohol is a diuretic.

Situation: Hoping to prevent cancer
Remedy: Make yourself a cup of hot chocolate. "Cocoa powder has more antioxidant power than green tea or any fruit or vegetable you can name," says Dr. Applegate. Numerous studies have shown that antioxidants fight cancer.

Situation: Stuck in the bathroom with diarrhea
Remedy: Diarrhea swiftly depletes the fluids and essential electrolytes that keep your system balanced. You need to replace them fast, so have a sports drink to refuel. Better yet, if you have Pedialyte in the house for your kids, try that. (Pedialyte also comes in freezer pops, in case you're having trouble keeping down fluids.)

Situation: Sick with an infection
Remedy: Green or black tea fights infections, even those caused by antibiotic-resistant bacteria. In lab studies, a component in the tea made *Staphylococcus aureus*—the resistant superbug—more vulnerable. Also, chicken soup appears to

have properties similar to penicillin's, and simply breathing in the vapors can open your sinuses.

Situation: Dinner's not for an hour, but you're famished now

Remedy: You need some fat and protein to feel satisfied, but you don't want to fill up. The perfect solution is 1 percent milk. "Pretzels or other snacks aren't satisfying enough, and heavier foods will dampen your appetite," explains Dr. Applegate.

Situation: Suffering from a headache

Remedy: Since your brain is three-quarters water, maybe dehydration is the problem. So first try 16 ounces of water. If you're suffering from a migraine, brew a pot of coffee. Caffeine has a constricting effect on the arteries in your head, which can help relieve pain.

Situation: Tired

Remedy: Pass on the caffeine and have a club soda with lemon or lime. The carbonation and aroma will energize you.

Situation: Hung over

Remedy: Drink a spicy V8 vegetable juice or a virgin Bloody Mary, suggests Paul Lachance, Ph.D., of Rutgers University. "The spices help dilate blood vessels, which could speed recovery by improving blood circulation." Also, antioxidants from the tomatoes will help fight damage from the alcohol.

Situation: Preparing for a workout

Remedy: Drink 17 ounces of water or a sports drink 2 hours before exercise, according to the American College of Sports Medicine. If your workout lasts longer than an hour, have a sports drink. Your fluid intake should match your sweat loss, and your drink should contain carbohydrates and electrolytes to help move water to your intestines.

Situation: Hoarse with a sore throat

Remedy: The vitamin C in orange juice would help, but the acid might exacerbate the soreness. So try tea with a few lemon wedges squeezed in—you'll get a dose of vitamin C, and the warmth will soothe your throat.

Situation: Trying to heal dry skin

Remedy: The next time you make a drink in the blender, toss in some flaxseed, suggests Dr. Applegate. The oil from this grain, which you can buy at supermarkets or health food stores, will help keep your skin smooth and glowing.

Situation: Thirsty and broke

Remedy: Switch from fancy bottled water to tap water. In a recent survey of the purity of bottled waters, one-third of 103 brands failed to meet either industry guidelines or state standards.

When Good Vegetables Taste Bad

Some of the healthiest foods are also the worst tasting. Follow these tips to make eating them easier on the palate.

Ask men which vegetables they hate most, and broccoli, brussels sprouts, beets, and spinach line up in a photo finish. Ask nutritionists which vegetables are best for you, and the same names show up in the top tier. Mother Nature is a practical joker. Some of the foods we most detest protect us the best.

We're not here to tell you to eat your vegetables—that's your mother's job. But we are here to make sure you know about all of life's tonics—even the less-than-delicious ones. Plain fact: If we listed all the ways these four vegetables can keep you well, you'd be reading until noon tomorrow.

You get dessert whether or not you eat your vegetables. But you get the health protection only if you're man enough to take the bitter with the sweet. We believe in seizing every single health opportunity out there, so we came up with some ways to maximize nutritional gain and minimize tastebud pain.

Broccoli
The antioxidants in broccoli limit the cellular damage caused by free radicals, and may have anti-inflammatory and antiviral properties as well. The top reason you should eat it: Broccoli is a powerful defender against cancer. "Broccoli bumps up the enzymes that rev up our systems to detoxify carcinogens," says Beverly Clevidence, Ph.D., a research nutritionist with the USDA.

To make it taste good:
- Skip the stalks. Broccoli florets have three times as much beta-carotene as the stems, and they're a great source of lutein, another potent antioxidant.
- Barbecue it. Throw some steamed broccoli and raw onions into one of those wire vegetable-barbecuing baskets, pour barbecue sauce over the mix, toss it, and grill it up over a low flame. Put some well-cooked meat on top for a few minutes, so some of the meat flavor drips into the vegetables. (Don't char either of them—some studies suggest that burnt foods contain carcinogens.)
- Stash it. The principle here: Hide broccoli in foods you like. At the last

minute, add steamed florets to the rattlesnake chili or your favorite canned soup. Whenever you have pizza, order broccoli as a topping. You won't even notice the cancer protection.

Brussels Sprouts

Nitrogen compounds called indoles protect you against colon cancer and lung cancer, and they may also cut your risk of prostate cancer. What's more, if a food fight erupts, sprouts make great ammo. They sting.

To make them taste good:

- Go small. Buy compact sprouts with a bright green color. They emit a less cabbagey odor when they're cooked.
- Skewer them. Boil brussels sprouts for a few minutes, then spear them and grill them with beef. Add barbecue sauce.
- Chop them. One problem with sprouts is their density. You bite into one and it's a little bomb of bitterness. So steam them until they're cooked, then chop them up and sneak them into soups or stews.
- Season them. You can hide the strong flavor of sprouts with zesty seasonings, such as mustard, caraway, sage, and garlic. Sauté steamed sprouts in a little olive oil with garlic. Then add a squeeze of lemon.

Beets

Beets are high in folate (folic acid), a vitamin that helps protect against heart disease, stroke, and colon cancer. They are also one of the best sources of anti-cancer antioxidants.

To make them taste good:

- Make them snack food. Cut beets into thin slices, top each with a dab of olive oil and fresh herbs and spices, and bake them on a cookie sheet for 30 to 60 minutes at 450°F. Baking intensifies beets' natural sweetness and locks in nutrients that are lost in the water if you boil them.

Spinach

One serving supplies nearly a full day's worth of vitamin A and half your vitamin C. Like beets, spinach is loaded with folate, and it also has two antioxidants that protect against macular degeneration, the leading cause of blindness in people over 65.

To make it taste good:
- Seek the skinny. At the market, look for thin stems. Spinach with thick stems is often bitter.
- Add a lasagna layer. Lasagna is so good, what with all the mozzarella and lean ground beef and tomato sauce and stuff, that you won't even notice a layer of spinach. Your body will, though. (Boil and drain the spinach first.)
- Do a sandwich switch. Use fresh spinach, not lettuce, on a meat or tuna sandwich.
- Try a Japanese salad. Dress your spinach salad with an Asian concoction made of ½ cup rice vinegar, 2 tablespoons fresh lemon juice, ¼ cup vegetable oil, 1½ teaspoons sesame oil, ½ teaspoon grated lemon zest, 3½ teaspoons soy sauce, 1 teaspoon Dijon mustard, ¼ teaspoon sugar, 2 teaspoons minced ginger, and a minced garlic clove. (This will make 1¼ cups. That's 10 two-tablespoon servings.)
- Whip up a stealth dip. Mix 10 ounces of cooked spinach with ½ cup nonfat sour cream, ½ cup plain fat-free yogurt, 1 cup finely chopped scallions, 1 can (8 ounces) finely chopped water chestnuts, salt, pepper, ground mustard, dried tarragon, and one crushed garlic clove. Chill and use as a dip or baked-potato topping.

Burgers for Better Health

The burger you choose could offer unexpected health benefits.

Health foods fall into one of two categories. There's the kind that might prevent cancer, if you could only bring yourself to eat it. Then there's the hamburger kind. They didn't start out as health food, they don't look like health food, and we guarantee they don't taste like health food, but the burgers below definitely act like health food. Make them a regular part of your diet, and they'll help lower your odds of developing heart disease and cancer, reduce your stress levels, put more meat on your muscles, cut your bathroom time, and rev up your sex life. Just mix up the ingredients, slap a patty on the grill, and let the healing begin.

The Muscle Burger

Building muscle is hard work. If you're weight training, your body needs an extra 16 grams of protein a day for every pound of muscle you want to pack on. This combo meal provides 42 grams of protein, about what you would find in two protein shakes. Top with romaine lettuce, tomato, and Swiss cheese. Use a whole wheat bun and add the fruit salad for extra calcium, magnesium, and potassium, to protect against muscle cramping.

Burger
>   8 ounces ground dark turkey meat
>   8 ounces extra-lean ground beef (97% fat-free)
>   4 egg whites
>   1 cup finely chopped mushrooms
>   2 teaspoons minced garlic

Makes 4 patties

Per burger: 334 calories, 38 grams protein, 23 grams carbohydrates, 12.5 grams fat (32% of calories), 121 milligrams cholesterol, 2 grams fiber, 400 milligrams sodium

Fruit Salad
>   ½ ounce almonds
>   1 diced apple
>   1 diced banana
>   2 tablespoons fat-free vanilla yogurt

The Longevity Burger

Eat too many cheeseburgers, and all that saturated fat could eventually raise your risk of prostate cancer. Eat these ultra-lean burgers, and you may help prevent the disease. Soy foods, such as tofu, can inhibit the growth of cancerous cells; the lycopene in the tomatoes may lower your risk of prostate cancer by as much as 35 percent; and a whole wheat bun contains the cancer-fighting mineral selenium. Top with reduced-fat mozzarella cheese, onion, and pizza sauce (more lycopene). Finish off your meal with a slice of watermelon, another good source of lycopene.

Burger
>   8 ounces extra-lean ground beef (97% fat-free)
>   8 ounces ground turkey breast
>   24 rehydrated sun-dried tomato halves, finely diced
>   1 cup soft, silken low-fat tofu, mashed fine
>   4 tablespoons tomato paste

2 teaspoons minced garlic
2 teaspoons dried basil

Makes 4 patties

Per burger: 391 calories, 45 grams protein, 41 grams carbohydrates, 9.2 grams fat (19% of calories), 109 milligrams cholesterol, 4 grams fiber, 723 milligrams sodium

The Heart Burger

Just one of these fish burgers contains 2 grams of omega-3 fatty acids. That's about half the amount you need to eat each week to lower your risk of heart disease by 25 percent, your blood pressure by an average of six points, and your heart rate by four beats per minute. Garlic does its part by helping to prevent the formation of blood clots. Top with Dijon-style mustard on a poppy or sesame seed bun. Add some sweet-potato chips, which are rich in beta-carotene and may also help reduce your risk of heart disease.

Burger
16 ounces canned salmon, flaked with a fork
4 garlic cloves, finely minced
2 small onions, finely chopped
2 teaspoons dried dill
4 egg whites

Makes 4 patties

Per burger: 346 calories, 32 grams protein, 30 grams carbohydrates, 10 grams fat (27% of calories), 62 milligrams cholesterol, 2 grams fiber, 992 milligrams sodium

The Libido Burger

This burger's complex carbohydrates will give you sexual staying power. Use a whole-grain pita for the bun and top with 1 tablespoon fat-free sour cream and some cucumber slices. The calcium in the sour-cream topping is necessary for the transmission of nerve signals. Add the spinach salad to maximize the effect: The mushrooms and sunflower seeds contain zinc, which may promote sperm production, and B vitamins, which are important for a healthy sex drive; the onions contain flavonoids to keep your blood flowing where you need it most.

Burger
   16 ounces extra-lean ground beef (97% fat-free)
   1 cup cooked brown rice
   2 teaspoons minced garlic
   2 teaspoons dried oregano

Makes 4 patties

Per burger: 328 calories, 36 grams protein, 48 grams carbohydrates, 4.2 grams fat (10% of calories), 120 milligrams cholesterol, 4 grams fiber, 247 milligrams sodium

Spinach Salad
   Raw spinach
   Fresh mushrooms
   ½ small onion, sliced
   ½ bell pepper, sliced
   1 ounce sunflower seeds

The Stress Burger

Feeling strung out? Reach for a turkey burger and top it with two slices of reduced-fat Cheddar cheese and some ketchup. Both turkey and cheese contain tryptophan, a chemical that is converted to serotonin in the brain. The more serotonin you have, the more relaxed you feel. A whole wheat bun will calm you with chromium and magnesium, two minerals necessary for counteracting stress hormones. Add the vegetable salad with red pepper and tomato for extra vitamin C to help build your body's supply of the stress-busting chemical dopamine.

Burger
   16 ounces ground turkey breast
   1 cup finely chopped onions

Makes 4 patties

Per burger: 402 calories, 41 grams protein, 31 grams carbohydrates, 12 grams fat (27% of calories), 96 milligrams cholesterol, 3 grams fiber, 924 milligrams sodium

Vegetable Salad
> Leaf lettuce
> ½ red bell pepper, diced
> 1 small tomato, diced
> ½ small onion, diced

The Fiber Burger

Your average quarter-pound burger contains about 2 grams of fiber, including what's in the bun, but when this bean burger is paired with a whole wheat bun, it tops out at about 10 grams. Add that much fiber to what you're already eating each day, and you can lower your cholesterol level by as much as 10 percent and reduce your risk of colon cancer by up to 33 percent. Top this spicy burger with a thick slice of onion and some salsa. To rack up even more fiber, pair your burger with some black-bean tortilla chips. Six chips provides 3 colon-clearing grams. Remember to open the windows.

Burger
> 16 ounces extra-lean ground beef (97% fat-free)
> 1 cup canned black beans, mashed with a fork
> 2–4 teaspoons chili powder
> 2 teaspoons minced garlic
> 4 tablespoons diced green chili peppers

Makes 4 patties

Per burger: 269 calories, 37 grams protein, 33 grams carbohydrates, 4.4 grams fat (12% of calories), 120 milligrams cholesterol, 7 grams fiber, 692 milligrams sodium

Flu-Fighting Foods

Arm yourself with these foods to boost your immunity during the next flu season.

Every year you get your flu shot, take your vitamin C, even try to follow your mother's advice and avoid leaving the house with a wet head or without pants. And every year that gets you the same thing: sick. Really sick.

What are you doing wrong? Probably nothing. You just need to start doing more things right. Like getting the most out of the most powerful flu-fighting, cold-killing weapon in your arsenal: your immune system. Just as what you eat can lower your risk of cancer and protect you from heart disease, putting the right foods on your plate can supercharge your immune system. So drop the bottle of echinacea and pick up the foods listed below; you have some eating to do.

Slurp some tomato soup for lunch. To beat back a cold, you slurp chicken noodle soup, but to avoid getting that cold in the first place, ladle out some tomato. In a study published in the *American Journal of Clinical Nutrition*, 10 subjects ate a tomato-rich diet for 3 weeks and a tomato-free diet for 3 more weeks. While subjects were on the tomato diet, their infection-fighting white blood cells sustained 38 percent less free-radical damage than when they ate no tomato products. Researchers speculate that the lycopene in tomatoes acts as an antioxidant, helping white blood cells resist the damaging effects of free radicals.

Snack on some yogurt. It has finally earned its reputation as a health food: A new study suggests that eating a container of yogurt daily helps prevent colds and flu. Researchers at the University of California at Davis had 60 people eat either 1 cup of yogurt with live cultures each day, 1 cup of pasteurized yogurt each day, or no yogurt at all. Over the course of a year, the people who ate either kind of yogurt had a lower incidence of coughing, colds, and wheezing.

Guzzle a sports drink during your workout. Not only will drinking a sports drink help your body recover from a punishing workout, but it may also protect you from the latest strain of the flu. According to a study published in the *International Journal of Sport Nutrition*, when 10 triathletes drank more than 1 cup of sports drink every 15 minutes during intense exercise, they had significantly better immune response than when they drank a placebo. Taking in more carbohydrates may prevent the normal exercise-induced rise in the body's levels of cortisol, an immune-suppressing hormone.

Add some red pepper. Mice that were given a daily dose of capsaicin—the compound that makes red peppers hot—had nearly three times more antibody-producing cells after 3 weeks than those given no capsaicin. More antibodies means fewer colds and infections. "Results of other studies suggest that eating food containing hot components such as capsaicin may improve immune status," says Rina Yu, Ph.D., of the University of Ulsan in Korea, the lead researcher.

Get nutty. Each Brazil nut contains about 100 micrograms of selenium, which, according to a study published in the *Archives of Internal Medicine*, may help prevent you from getting your yearly respiratory infection. Researchers gave 725 elderly subjects either a supplement containing vitamins A, C, and E; a mineral supplement containing 100 micrograms of selenium; a combination of the two; or a placebo every day for 2 years. Over the course of the study, those subjects who took the straight mineral supplement had fewer respiratory infections than the rest. "A deficiency of selenium can hinder your body's disease-fighting performance," says Ashini Shah, R.D., of the New England Medical Center in Boston. You can buy Brazil nuts in most supermarkets and health-food stores.

Think "low," not "no." Keeping your fat intake low will keep both your heart and your immune system healthy. "It was found that putting human volunteers on a low-fat diet, at about 25 percent of total calories, increased the effectiveness of their immune cells," says Philip Calder, Ph.D., professor of human nutrition at the University of Southampton in England. But don't think that cutting out even more fat is better. "A very low fat intake, less than 10 percent of calories, might result in a deficiency of omega-3 and omega-6 fatty acids, which can markedly impair the body's ability to make new cells to combat infections," warns Dr. Calder.

The Vanity Diet

If you want to look better, you can pay for plastic surgery—or you can simply eat better. Here are some suggestions to get you started.

Dog food has a lot going for it. Just read the label: It promises bright eyes, a glossy coat, strong teeth. If your mutt eats this chow, he'll take Best of Show and score with the bitches. But what about human chow? Sure, the right foods will help us dodge heart disease and cancer, but what about our eyes, coat, and teeth? Why can't we eat to improve our looks?

We can. After much pointless snacking, we brushed the chocolate jimmies from our laps and dialed up the nutrition experts. They tipped us off about a bunch of foods that do plenty for the appearance of the average biped. How about eating grapes to grow hair? Or an apricot to help keep your skin supple? Heck, you can even eat meat—not horse meat—to lose your gut. Here's a list of the links between good taste and good looks. No need to eat from a bowl on the floor.

Binge on bagels for bigger muscles. If you keep leaving the gym with the same muscles you came in with, you're probably short on carbohydrates. Without enough carbohydrates, you won't have the stamina you need at the end of your workout. "Muscle growth happens during those tough last reps, when your muscles tear and repair themselves," says Debra Wein, R.D., a nutritionist and exercise expert in Boston. "In fact, during intense weight lifting, your body is using carbohydrates exclusively." Aim for at least 3 to 5 grams of carbohydrates per pound of body weight daily.

Boost your broccoli intake for perfect posture. To prevent osteoporosis and the resulting Quasimodofication of your back, you need plenty of calcium. For men, that means at least four servings a day of dairy products such as low-fat milk, cheese, or yogurt. But calcium isn't the only mineral you need. Magnesium also lays down new bone structure, according to Judith Petry, M.D., a nutritionist in Vermont. Good sources include brown rice, spinach, and broccoli. Wash it all down with at least one 8-ounce glass of water to ensure that both minerals are absorbed.

Eat an apricot to stop dry skin. Why slather on your wife's apricot-scented lotion when you can eat the real thing and prevent dry skin from the inside out? According to Richard Glogau, M.D., professor of dermatology at the University of California at San Francisco, it's the vitamin A in apricots that does the trick. "Vitamin A helps your body manufacture more keratin, a substance that protects the skin from the elements," he says. Carrots, cantaloupes, and sweet potatoes are also high in vitamin A. Avoid megadose supplements.

Guzzle a bottle of water to banish baggy eyes. Think of your eyes as your body's water gauge. When the tissues around them are puffy and swollen, you can bet that the well is almost dry. Guys who hang out in air-conditioned offices should be drinking at least a quart of water per day. If you spend your days sweating away in a coal mine, drink more. It doesn't have to be water; most other fluids are just as good, except one: "Alcohol is known to deplete intercellular fluids," says Dr. Petry. You don't want that to happen. Avoid the sunken look in your eyes by cutting down on bar-stool time.

Order a steak sandwich to lose your gut. You may be able to curb your appetite by eating more foods rich in zinc. In a study published in the *Journal of the American College of Nutrition,* researchers found that an increase in zinc consumption caused a rise in leptin, a hormone that controls body fat by telling you when you've had enough to eat. Your body takes an increase in leptin as a signal to build muscle instead of store fat. Lean red meats and whole grains are rich in zinc. To us, that sounds like a Philly steak (hold the cheese) on a whole wheat bun.

Grab a bunch of grapes to thicken your hair. To win the war against baldness, you need to beat dihydrotestosterone (DHT), a hormone that halts your hair follicles' growth cycle. And the best defense against DHT may be grape seeds. Japanese researchers discovered that when bald mice were treated topically with grape-seed extract, it stimulated their hair-growth cycle in a manner similar to minoxidil, a.k.a. Rogaine. Credit for the results goes to plant compounds called proanthocyanidins.

Okay, you're not a bald mouse. But it couldn't hurt to take a supplement containing grape-seed extract, or include more red grape juice and red grapes in your diet.

Slice some peppers to prevent scars. If you've suffered a nasty cut, make red bell peppers part of your treatment plan. The extra vitamin C will enhance the performance of tissue-building amino acids, which in turn will help prevent your gash from healing as an unsightly scar. "Vitamin C is critical to the healing process and especially scar formation," says Chris Rosenbloom, Ph.D., R.D., a professor of nutrition at Georgia State University in Atlanta. Other foods high in vitamin C include kiwis, grapefruit juice, and cranberry juice.

Think vitamin E to wrinkle-proof your face. You already know that using sunscreen now will help prevent creases on your face at 50. What you may not know is that you can buy extra insurance for your mug with vitamin E. This antioxidant helps to combat wrinkle-causing free-radical damage. "Vitamin E will help a sunburn heal faster if your body is stocked up on it," says Cindy Moore, R.D., of the American Dietetic Association. In addition to eating avocados, sunflower seeds, and whole grains, you can take a daily supplement containing 200 international units.

Drink OJ to protect your teeth. Before you brush and floss, pour and swig some calcium-fortified orange juice. You'll get two mouth guards in one: calcium and vitamin C. Researchers at the State University of New York at Buffalo studied nearly 15,000 people and found that those who took in less than 500 milligrams of calcium a day were at a higher risk for tooth loss caused by gum disease. Calcium is believed to strengthen the jawbone against the bacteria that cause gum disease, and the vitamin C in OJ may help strengthen gum tissue.

Dine and Drive

If you usually get your three squares behind the wheel, here's how to fill your tank.

Men love to drive. And we love to eat. Our idea of a concept car is one with twin turbochargers, cupholders that work, and a glove compartment that doubles as a microwave oven. Sadly, eating while driving is dangerous—to other drivers, your belly, and worst of all, your upholstery. Once you drip taco sauce on your leather-trimmed interior, you'll have to learn to live with it, or sell the car.

So how do you manage in-car meals with your suit, weight, and life intact? You heed the advice—as we did—of the hardened highwaymen who spend most of their eating hours behind the wheel. "I think of every minute I park as a mile lost," says Dale Salsbury, a veteran trucker who's been eating his three squares on 18 wheels since 1962. And just to make sure that none of our advisory board of truckers and traveling salesmen took a wrong turn at the drive-thru, we asked for directions—a first!—from Jackie Newgent, R.D., a spokeswoman for the American Dietetic Association.

So this is your map and your menu. Follow the directions faithfully and you'll never again need to loosen your seat belt after a meal. Nor will you have to convince your wife that the stain on the back seat really is just special sauce.

The Morning Commute

Drink your Wheaties. Cereal is one tough customer; after you puree it in a blender with milk and fruit, it'll still hit you with the same nutritional punch. Mix a batch, refrigerate it, and fill a spill-proof mug anytime.

One blend to try:

½ cup All-Bran extra fiber cereal
1 cup fat-free milk
½ cup blueberries
1 tablespoon honey

Dump all of the ingredients into a blender and puree. You'll get 17 grams of fiber, 13 grams of protein, calcium from the milk, and antioxidants from the blueberries—the richest fruit source. Note: Nutrition totals may be slightly less with Cocoa Krispies.

Make a fruit roll-up. What are pancakes without the syrup, the butter, and the sausage on the side? Healthy and exponentially easier to eat in the car. Wrap two hotcakes around a peeled banana and you'll cut the calories and fat in half while taking in more than 80 grams of carbohydrates, 10 grams of protein, and the potassium necessary to help turn it all into energy. And don't toss the banana peel. When you get to work, rub the inside of the peel on your shoes for a quick shine.

Squeeze some yogurt. Normally, eating yogurt on four wheels is a two-hand operation. But not for John Powers, a Colorado-based dry goods hauler. He swears by Yoplait Go-Gurt, tubes of squeezable yogurt. Two Go-Gurts and a bagel have more than 17 grams of protein, 80 grams of carbohydrates, and 30 percent of your Daily Value (DV) of calcium. Flavors include Strawberry Splash, Berry Blue Blast, Strawberry Banana Burst, and Watermelon Meltdown. Our proposed new flavor: Orange Orgasm.

Make the fastest (and healthiest) breakfast sandwich to go. Ready in less than 2 minutes.

1 slice low-fat American cheese
½ teaspoon trans fat–free margarine (trans fatty acids increase your risk of heart disease)
2 slices (2 ounces) Canadian bacon (much less fat than the American kind)
1 omega-3 fatty acid fortified egg (look in the dairy case; they may help lower your risk of heart disease)
1 Thomas's English Muffin, Honey Wheat (may help reduce your cholesterol levels)

Split the muffin, toast it, and add margarine. Break the egg into a microwavable dish, prick the yolk with a toothpick, and cover with plastic wrap. Cook on high for 30 seconds, cover, and let stand for 30 seconds. Start with the bottom half of the English muffin, then add cheese, egg, and bacon, and top with the other muffin half. Nuke for 20 more seconds, wrap in foil, and toss in your car. For an authentic fast-food experience, don't give yourself any napkins.

Pick up a tart who's ready to strip. Here's one breakfast-food gimmick that works: Pop Tarts perforated to break into three easy-to-manage strips. They're called Pop Tarts Snak-Stix and they come ready to travel in a resealable plastic bag. Three strips have 37 grams of carbohydrates, plus some B vitamins, magnesium, calcium, and zinc, and just 5 grams of fat.

A Traffic Jam

Pull out a bag of fruit. Dried fruit is driver-friendly fruit: There's nothing to peel, drip down your sleeve, or spoil. Even better, it's concentrated nutrition. A half cup of dried prunes, apricots, pears, and apples has about 8 grams of fiber and 64 grams of carbohydrates, plus ellagic acid and bioflavonoids—phytochemicals that may help prevent cancer and heart disease.

Hide some Easter eggs. Keep a stash of quick protein within arm's reach by bringing along a couple of hard-boiled eggs. Peel one while the babe in front of you is checking her makeup. Each contains 6 grams of protein, selenium, and lutein, a phytochemical that may help reduce the risk of colon cancer. Rotten-egg watch: They'll keep for only a few hours, so you can't save any for the return trip. But you can still juggle with them.

Bite the head off a giraffe. Or a leg off a lion. Either way, eating animal crackers can satisfy your sadistic streak and your hunger. "They're low-fat and fairly filling, and there's no mess. Sometimes I buy a 5-pound bag at Sam's Club," says John Powers. Twenty-five crackers (about one box) have 42 grams of carbohydrates, 4 grams of protein, and 8 grams of fat, most of which is the monounsaturated kind, which can improve your ratio of good-to-bad cholesterol.

Chew on this. Like some kind of teething Rottweiler, you gnaw and you gnaw on beef jerky. For what? About 160 calories and 4 grams of saturated fat in just two strips. You're better off with Jack Link's Kippered Beef Steak. One ounce has 12 grams of protein but just 75 calories and less than half a gram of saturated fat.

Say cheese. Finally, a situation to justify the existence of string cheese. Buy the Healthy Choice mozzarella or Cheddar variety for a very low-fat and very portable source of protein and calcium. A recent study showed that eating more dairy sources of calcium may inhibit weight gain by increasing the breakdown of body fat and decreasing its formation.

Rush Hour

Hit a chicken shack. There's a tidier way to pick up meat on the road than stopping for asphalt-baked venison: Buy some drumsticks. Each comes with a free commuter handle and, if you buy KFC's tender-roast variety, that's just 97 calories, 4 grams of fat, and practically zero grease.

Show up on Dave's doorstep. You won't find fast food that's healthy and mobile on the menu; you have to ask for it. Here's what to say at Wendy's: "I'll have one Chicken Caesar Pita, hold the cheese and dressing, and go easy on the vegetables." What you'll get is less fat and calories and a whopping 34 grams of protein, 47 grams of carbohydrates, 4 grams of fiber, and close to 50 percent of your DV for vitamin A. Oh yeah, and ask why is it that Wendy looks like Ronald McDonald's illegitimate daughter. They'll like that.

Run into a Blimpie or hop on the Subway. Both sub shops offer half-foot turkey and half-foot roast beef subs that have between 4 and 5 grams of total fat (minus the mayo). But while Blimpie slices its rolls straight through, Subway cuts theirs in a V. "When the bread is cut like that, you end up wearing more than you eat," says Dale Salsbury. To further minimize your mess, hold the oil and vinegar.

Eat Chinese food—with one hand. Only one Chinese food is truly road-worthy: egg rolls. They come sealed in their own containers and, if you buy the large, frozen kind, have only 107 calories and 2 grams of fat each. Eat three and you've just had a meal with 54 grams of carbohydrates, 9 grams of protein, 3 grams of fiber, plus 25 percent of your DV of folate, a vitamin that may help prevent heart disease.

Have a pie for dinner. Little Caesar's and Domino's have smaller slices than the mom-and-pop places, and the inflexible crusts are topped with cheese and sauce that stays put. Order either a plain cheese pie or one with green peppers from Little Caesar's, or a Domino's thin crust with onions. They're all lower in fat than other choices, and the tomato sauce and onions both contain phytochemicals that may help prevent cancer.

More Tips for Road Warriors

Don't die over spilled milk. Staying slim and clean doesn't count for much if you end up eating the guardrail for dessert. Here's how to survive a meal on the street.

- It's not just rude to talk while eating; it's also dangerous. If the cell phone chirps, put the chips down.
- Set the cruise control to the speed limit. You won't have to worry about working the pedal and watching for state troopers in the bushes.
- Keep your free hand on the wheel. "When I'm eating, I usually keep my left hand at about 9 or 10 o'clock on the steering wheel," says Ernie Douglas, a Wyoming-based truck driver. "That's where you have the most control."
- Never take your eyes off the road to handle food. Always keep it within arm's reach in the same place.
- Never eat anything greasy. Your hand may slip off the wheel when you suddenly try to swerve to hit—er . . . miss a cat crossing the road.
- Never drive with your knees.

- Use an accordion-style straw. This way you won't be tilting your head back to chug some Mountain Dew at the exact moment that Granny nods off and slides into your lane.
- Avoid juice boxes and other puncture-the-packaging-with-a-straw beverages. They're difficult enough to manage when you have both hands free.

Pass a spot inspection. If you eat in the car, you'll need a spot remover. Peter Calcandy, who has splattered ties from Long Island to Chicago, recommends dry-cleaning solvents called 1ne and 2wo (pronounced one and two; clever, eh?). "2wo is great for getting mayonnaise spots off your necktie," he says. "Works great on upholstery, too." 1ne is good for syrup, ketchup, and coffee spots. Call (609) 799-3312 to order. They cost about $7 each.

Use the best coffee mug on the planet. We subjected a bunch of mugs and tumblers to tips, drops, and the occasional Hail Mary pass. We liked the Absolutely SpillProof Tumbler ($25) because it kept the coffee how we like it: hot and off our pants. It also has a neat lid that you can slide open with one hand. You can buy one at specialty coffee shops or through Sharper Image, (800) 344-5555. The best feature: no references to Seattle.

Avoid nasty spills. Even the most nimble car jockeys occasionally hit a pot hole and give up the Big Gulp. Fortunately, there's the Drive Time Dribble Bib, with a terry-cloth side to absorb up to 2 ounces of liquid, and a plastic backing to prevent seepage. The price? $9.95 and the mockery of toll-booth attendants. Call (800) 259-0894, or visit www.dribblebib.com.

Wrap it up the night before. Mexican food has its place in the car—usually on the upholstery. But not if you make your own with a soft tortilla shell. It won't crumble like bread, and if you wrap it the right way, it will keep all but the most fluid ingredients off your lap. Look for whole wheat tortillas (Mission Foods makes them) and pack 'em with healthy stuffings like shredded turkey, low-fat cheese, diced tomatoes, green peppers, and onions.

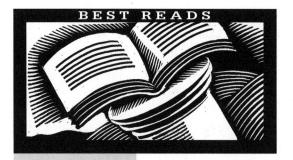

BEST READS

Stick-to-Your-Ribs Sides

Baked. Mashed. Fried. That pretty much sums up your options for spuds, right? Wrong. As Don Mauer shows in the following recipes from his book, A Guy's Guide to Great Eating *(Houghton Mifflin), potatoes don't have to be fried in lard or smothered in sour cream to taste good. Read on for some recipes for potatoes and other side dishes that manage to have big flavor without a lot of fat.*

For satisfaction on a plate, nothing beats a mound of whipped potatoes or an aromatic square of warm corn bread. With side dishes like these, you'll never have to worry about leaving the table hungry.

Unlike traditional versions, these accompaniments don't get their flavor from gobs of butter or sour cream. My Special Mashed Potatoes have uncommon flavor notes and are unbelievably low in fat. They're cooked in a mixture of fat-free chicken broth, white wine, and sautéed onions, with finely chopped good-quality black olives stirred in at the end.

Rice can be as satisfying as potatoes, especially if you choose jasmine rice, which is particularly aromatic. When it simmers, it gives off a scent that reminds me of popcorn, and it has a flavor that ordinary white rice can't approach.

Special Mashed Potatoes

My brother Tom, who is a chef, created these special potatoes. Cooking them in chicken broth and white wine with sautéed onions gives complex flavors to the dish that plain water never could.

1½ teaspoons unsalted butter
½ yellow onion, finely chopped
2 pounds Yukon Gold potatoes, peeled and cut into ¼-inch-thick slices
4 cups fat-free reduced-sodium chicken broth
¼ cup dry white wine

¾ teaspoon salt
¼ teaspoon fresh-ground black pepper
¼ cup kalamata olives, pitted and minced

Melt the butter in a 5-quart saucepan over medium heat. Add the onion and sauté until translucent, 3 to 4 minutes; do not let brown. Add the potatoes, broth, and wine and bring to a boil. Reduce the heat to low and simmer for 15 to 20 minutes, or until the potatoes can be easily pierced with a knife. Place a colander in a large bowl and pour the potato mixture into the colander; reserve the liquid.

Place the potatoes in a large mixing bowl. With an electric mixer on low, begin to break up the potatoes, then increase the speed to medium and mix for 1 to 2 minutes more, until the potatoes start to become smooth. Add ¾ cup of the reserved cooking liquid, salt, and pepper and mix until smooth and creamy, about 2 minutes. If the potatoes seem stiff or dry, add up to ¼ cup more cooking liquid.

Stir in the olives by hand and serve.

Makes 4 servings
Per serving: 245 calories (9.3% from fat), 2.6 g fat (0.9 g saturated fat), 3.8 g protein, 49 g carbohydrate, 4 mg cholesterol, 597 mg sodium.
Cooking tip: Overmixing the potatoes will make them gummy. So will using a food processor.
Salt sense: Omitting the salt will reduce the sodium to 197 mg per serving.

Steakhouse Oven-Fried Potatoes

These steakhouse-style potatoes are cut in large rectangles and seasoned just right. They emerge from the oven golden brown on the outside and soft and sweet inside. I love to serve them with grilled flank steak and one of my creamy cabbage slaws.

1½ tablespoons olive oil
2 large garlic cloves, minced
1 teaspoon salt
½ teaspoon fresh-ground black pepper
4 8-ounce red-skin potatoes, scrubbed
Paprika to taste

Place the oven rack in the lower-middle position and preheat the oven to 425 degrees.

Place the oil, garlic, salt, and pepper in a large mixing bowl and whisk until combined.

Cut the potatoes into finger-size lengths ½-inch thick, 1 inch wide and as long as the potato. Pat the pieces dry with paper towels. Add them to the mixing bowl and toss until coated with oil.

Place the potatoes on a jelly-roll pan, making certain they do not touch each other. Sprinkle generously with the paprika. Bake for 15 minutes. Turn the potatoes and sprinkle generously with paprika. Bake for 15 minutes more, or until golden, and serve.

Makes 4 servings
Per serving: 229 calories (20.3% from fat), 5.1 g fat (0.7 g saturated fat), 3.8 g protein, 44.1 g carbohydrate, 0 mg cholesterol, 547 mg sodium.
Cooking tip: Lining the jelly-roll pan with heavy-duty foil makes for quick and easy cleanup.
Salt sense: Omitting the salt reduces the sodium to 14 mg per serving.

Zesty Curried Rice Pilaf

Thanks to the curry powder, this pilaf has such a stand-out flavor that I serve it with meats that are not highly seasoned, such as roast beef or turkey breast. A slightly sweet vegetable, such as steamed peas or carrots, goes well with it. The spiciness of curry powder is determined by the amount of hot pepper it contains. I keep several different brands on my spice rack.

1½ cups basmati rice
1 tablespoon butter
1 medium onion, chopped
1 tablespoon hot curry powder
⅛ teaspoon cayenne pepper
2½ cups fat-free reduced-sodium chicken broth (preferably homemade)
½ teaspoon salt
3 tablespoons chopped fresh parsley leaves

Place the rice in a medium bowl and cover with cold water. Stir the water around to remove the starch coating on the rice. Drain and continue washing and draining until the water is clear. Add enough warm water to cover the rice by 1 inch. Soak for 20 minutes. Drain.

After the rice has soaked for 15 minutes, place a medium nonstick saucepan over medium heat and add the butter. When it foams, add the onion and cook, stirring, for 5 minutes, or until softened. Add the drained rice and stir until coated with butter. Add the curry powder and cayenne pepper and cook, stirring, for 1 minute, or until fragrant.

Add the broth and salt to the saucepan and bring to a boil. Reduce the heat to low; cover and simmer until the rice is tender and the liquid is absorbed, about 17 minutes.

Remove from the heat and let stand, covered, for 5 minutes. Add the parsley and fluff the rice with a fork. Serve.

Makes 6 servings
Per serving: 204 calories (10.5% from fat), 2.4 g fat (1.9 g saturated fat), 4 g protein, 40.8 g carbohydrate, 5 mg cholesterol, 366 mg sodium.
Salt sense: Omitting the salt reduces the sodium to 188 mg per serving.

Fancy Sweet Corn Bread

This may be the best corn bread I've ever tasted. The buttermilk is essential, adding a sweet, tangy note that sets this quick bread apart.

1½ cups yellow cornmeal, preferably stone ground
½ cup unbleached all-purpose flour
3 tablespoons granulated sugar
2 teaspoons baking powder
½ teaspoon baking soda
1 large egg yolk
2 teaspoons canola oil
2 large egg whites
1½ cups low-fat buttermilk

Place the oven rack in the center, place an 8-by-8-by-2-inch baking pan on the rack and preheat the oven to 425 degrees.

In a medium mixing bowl, stir together the cornmeal, flour, sugar, baking powder, and baking soda. Set aside.

In a large mixing bowl, whisk together the egg yolk and oil until combined. Add the egg whites and buttermilk and whisk until combined. Add the cornmeal mixture and stir until just moistened; the batter will not be smooth.

Carefully remove the preheated pan from the oven and place it on a heatproof surface. Lightly spray the pan with vegetable oil. Immediately pour the batter into the pan, smooth the top, and bake for 25 minutes, or until the top is light brown and a toothpick inserted in the center comes out clean. Cool slightly and serve.

Makes 6 servings
Per serving: 229 calories (17.7% from fat), 4.5 g fat (0.6 g saturated fat), 6.7 g protein, 40.3 g carbohydrate, 36 mg cholesterol, 283 mg sodium.
Lean suggestions: When whisking in the buttermilk, you can add one of the following to the batter: ½ cup fresh or frozen whole-kernel yellow corn, or ½ cup grated reduced-fat sharp Cheddar cheese, or ¼ cup chopped onion and ¼ cup chopped green bell pepper or 1 chopped jalapeño.

For a Carolina flavor boost, substitute 2 teaspoons bacon grease for the 2 teaspoons canola oil.

Plain corn bread may be served with apple butter or strawberry preserves.

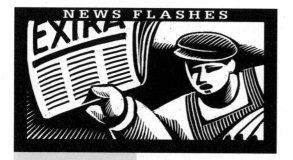

Stress at Lunchtime Could Equal Higher Cholesterol Levels

PARIS—Wolfing down your lunch at your desk might be efficient, but it definitely isn't healthy. Eating under stress can cause a dangerous spike in your cholesterol levels. When French researchers had people eat meals under various conditions, they found that cholesterol and triglyceride levels increased, and in some cases doubled, when the people were most stressed. "Stress slows down the rate at which fats are broken down, causing them to stay in the bloodstream longer," says Jean Dallongeville, M.D., Ph.D., the lead researcher. Since these fluctuations can increase the risk of heart disease, keeping your stress levels in check during mealtimes could be a matter of life and death.

For More Energy, Get Your Vitamin C

TEMPE, Ariz.—Take a lesson from English sailors: Suck on a citrus fruit before you do any real work. If you take in too little vitamin C (and there's roughly a 1-in-4 chance that you do), it can cause a dip in your energy levels. Researchers at Arizona State University noticed this connection when nine vitamin

C–depleted people underwent treadmill tests. After taking 500-milligram vitamin C supplements daily for 2 weeks, they were able to walk 10 percent faster. "Vitamin C may help your body metabolize fat for energy," says Carol Johnston, Ph.D., the study leader. Taking in the Recommended Dietary Allowance of 120 milligrams is easy: Just drink a cup of orange juice.

Cinnamon Identified as Bacteria Killer

MANHATTAN, Kans.—Roadside apple cider became notorious when it was linked to an outbreak of *Escherichia coli* bacteria. If that hasn't deterred you from buying a jug, you may at least want to add some cinnamon. A recent study showed that cinnamon kills *E. coli*. Kansas State University researchers contaminated 64-ounce containers of apple cider with *E. coli*, then added cinnamon. After 24 hours, 1 teaspoon of cinnamon had reduced the *E. coli* to undetectable levels.

Soybean Oil May Benefit Your Heart

BETHESDA, Md.—Eating soybean oil may lower your risk of dying of a heart attack. In a study published in the *American Journal of Clinical Nutrition*, researchers studied 76,283 people and found that those who ate five to six servings of soybean-oil–based salad dressing per week had one-sixth the rate of cardiac death of those who ate one serving or less. "Soybean oil is high in alpha-linoleic acid, which may help prevent clogged arteries and correct irregular heartbeats," says Frank Hu, M.D., Ph.D., the lead study author. Try to eat 1 to 2 tablespoons of a dressing made with soybean oil each day.

Olive Oil Linked to Lower Risk for Arthritis

ATHENS, Greece—Researchers in Greece report that eating olive oil may reduce your risk of arthritis. When the diets of 333 subjects were evaluated, researchers found that those who consumed olive oil most often had a 62 percent lower risk of rheumatoid arthritis than those who ate it infrequently. "The oleic acid in olive oil may combat the inflammatory changes that contribute to rheumatoid arthritis," says Athena Linos, M.D., the lead study author. To get these benefits and improve your good-to-bad cholesterol ratio, substitute olive oil for a few of the other fats in your diet at least every other day.

Pepper May Increase Absorption of Nutrients

FULTON, Md.—Break out the peppermill: Adding pepper to your meals may make them more nutritious. Researchers are finding that piperine, a phytochemical in pepper, may give you more bang for your broccoli. Spices like pepper accelerate the body's absorption of some nutrients, says James Duke, Ph.D., author of *The Green Pharmacy.* "I add pepper generously to my soups and salads," he says. It may take a lot of pepper to see the effect. But one company has been granted a patent on a process that extracts piperine from pepper, so a pill may be coming.

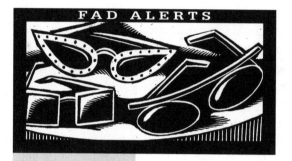

Eggs Fortified with Omega-3 Fatty Acids

Three companies—Eggland's Best, Gold Circle Farms, and Rose Acre Farms—offer eggs that are high in omega-3's. What's the benefit? Eating omega-3 fatty acids may help fight heart disease and depression. There's also a theory that taking in more omega-3's can lower your risk of Alzheimer's disease and inflammatory diseases, such as arthritis. In a Dutch study, subjects who ate one serving of omega-3–rich fish per week were 70 percent less likely to develop Alzheimer's than those who ate no fish.

Experts recommend getting 300 to 400 milligrams of omega-3's per day, which is about two eggs' worth.

Heart Bar

Advertisements for the Heart Bar ($2 each) claim that eating one a day can improve circulation and even relieve chest pain if you have heart disease. The active ingredient is 3 grams of L-arginine, an amino acid that dilates blood vessels. Taking a daily dose of about 500 milligrams of arginine has been shown to help men with arterial heart disease, but not those with damaged valves or enlarged heart tissue, says George Sopko, M.D., a cardiologist in Bethesda, Maryland. If your doctor thinks you should take arginine, he may recommend pills rather than a 180-calorie energy bar that's both gritty and mealy. Taking 500 milligrams a day in pill form would cost $30 a year. Eating 365 Heart Bars would run you $730—and add 27 pounds to your gut.

Kellogg's Ensemble with Psyllium

Many studies suggest that daily consumption of psyllium reduces cholesterol levels. Based on these findings, Kellogg's has developed a line of products under the brand name of Ensemble. The line includes breads, frozen entrees, pastas, cereals, desserts, and snacks fortified with the dietary fiber psyllium. A study published in the *American Journal of Clinical Nutrition* found that one dose of psyllium per day helped to lower total cholesterol levels by 7 percent and LDL cholesterol by 15 percent. "Dozens of studies show that psyllium is effective," confirms Clare Hasler, Ph.D., of the University of Illinois. In general, look for psyllium products that contain at least 1.7 grams of soluble fiber per serving.

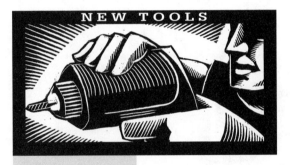

NEW TOOLS

Better Snacking

Spicy Steak Fries

Twenty chicken wings have 140 grams of fat. Munch on them as you watch the Monday night game, and you'll end up shaped like a football. Instead, try these low-fat, spicy steak fries.

5 medium potatoes (2 pounds)
¼ teaspoon salt
¼ teaspon pepper
⅛ teaspoon onion powder
1 crushed garlic clove, or 1 tablespoon garlic powder
1 tablespoon olive oil

Preheat the oven to 450°F. Peel the potatoes and cut each one lengthwise into six wedges. Place the potato wedges flat in a baking dish coated with nonstick spray. Sprinkle them with the salt, pepper, onion powder, garlic, and oil, then stir them around. Bake for 30 minutes or until they're brown.

Makes 6 servings
Per serving: 204 calories, 2 g fat (10% of calories), 43 g carbohydrates.

Healthier Version of a Popular Drink

Yoo-Hoo Lite

Regular Yoo-Hoo has just 1 gram of fat and 260 calories, so who needs the Lite stuff? Maybe you, if you want to cut the calories in half. The Lite is a bit thinner and sweeter than regular Yoo-Hoo, but it still has a rich chocolate flavor and the same puny gram of fat. Either drink will deliver 10 percent of your Daily Value for calcium.

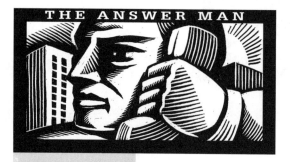

THE ANSWER MAN

The Lowdown on Joe

I know I should drink at least eight 8-ounce glasses of water per day. Does coffee count toward that total?
—B. C., Fargo, N.D.

A little. Coffee (as well as other caffeine-containing beverages such as tea and cola) has a mild diuretic effect, so your body retains less fluid from a cup of coffee than from a cup of water, says Craig Horswill, Ph.D., senior research scientist at the Gatorade Exercise Physiology Lab in Barrington, Illinois. You can count each 8 ounces of coffee you drink as half a glass of water. That means you'd have to drink a gallon of java every day to equal eight glasses of water. Eight glasses of water would generate just as many trips to the john, but it's sure easier on your stomach and nerves.

Topping Off the Protein Tank

Is there a limit to how much protein the body can digest at one time? I drink a protein supplement after my workout, but I'm afraid that the protein may be going to waste or, worse, is being stored as fat.
—T. L., Ft. Lauderdale

Weight lifters often focus too much on protein: They spend way too much time trying to calculate exactly how much they should eat, though most already take in more than they need, says Debra Wein, M.S., R.D., a Massachusetts nutritionist and a weight lifter herself. "There doesn't appear to be a strict limit on how much protein you can digest in one sitting," Wein says, "but we do know there's a limit to what the body can handle in a day." For most lifters, that's 0.5 to 0.6 gram of protein per pound of body weight. So if you weigh 170 pounds, you're looking at 85 grams to 102 grams per day. If you regularly consume more than that, you're setting yourself up for dehydration and strain on your kidneys, and the excess calories may be stored as fat.

Exactly when you eat your protein is up to you, but research suggests you're better off spreading it over the day than gulping it down in one shot. "Eating a little protein at each meal can help prevent food cravings, and there's reason to believe it's more readily available when the body needs it," says Wein.

The Morning After

When I drink dark beers, I don't get a hangover. But when I drink lighter-colored beers, I wake up feeling like Dean Martin after a bender. What gives?
—J. S., Massapequa, N.Y.

Blame it on carbonation, since most light-colored beers have more bubbles. "Carbonation increases the rate of alcohol absorption into the bloodstream," explains William Shoemaker, Ph.D., a professor at the University of Connecticut Alcohol Research Center and the school of medicine. "You've seen people drink champagne at weddings and start giggling within 30 seconds—it's a pharmacological effect." Since alcohol hits your system more quickly with a highly carbonated beer, and your liver works at a set pace, to reduce your hangover you should stretch the same amount of brew over more hours. Or drink less.

Form and Function

Can my body distinguish between the vitamins I get with my food and those I swallow in pill form?
—R. C., Richmond, Va.

Nope. "Supplements often have the same chemical composition as the vitamins in food," says Susan Adams, R.D., a spokeswoman for the American Dietetic

Association. But that doesn't mean food and pills work equally well in providing health benefits. "Other ingredients in foods can enhance or hinder the absorption of a particular nutrient," says Adams. The vitamin D in a glass of milk, for example, aids in the absorption of calcium. But compounds called oxalates make the calcium found in spinach more difficult to absorb.

The real concern: If you get your health by the pill, you'll miss out on the fiber and phytochemicals that fruits and vegetables provide. And that means eating more and more pills.

Melting Cheese with Ease

How can I keep my low-fat cheese from turning to rubber in the microwave?
—T. J., Detroit

To prevent this, spritz your nachos with a quick blast of cooking spray, such as Pam, before putting them in the microwave, or spray the inside of a grilled-cheese sandwich before you toss it in the pan. This adds just enough fat to make the cheese stay creamy when it melts.

If you're craving full-fat cheese for sandwiches or other meals, go easy on hard varieties. "Popular cheeses like Cheddar and mozzarella are the ones highest in fat," says Susan Swadener, Ph.D., instructor of food science and nutrition at California Polytechnic State University in San Luis Obispo. The gooey white cheeses like feta and low-fat cream cheese are usually lower in fat.

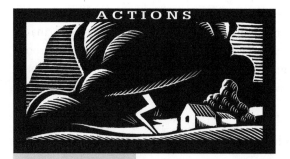

ACTIONS

Two-thirds of Americans—more of them men than women—say they're confused by news reports about what foods to avoid. It's no wonder. It seems like every time you turn on the TV or open the newspaper, there's some new report about the hidden fat lurking in yet another seemingly innocent food. What's a hungry guy to do?

First of all, use common sense. It should come as no surprise that a baked potato topped with, say, low-fat tomato salsa is better for you than french fries cooked in lard. And while a diet of french fries and chocolate pie certainly isn't going to improve your health, realize that a lot of foods *do* offer terrific health bonuses. From salmon for fighting heart disease to tomatoes for preventing cancer, wise food choices will strengthen and nourish you, not just fill you up. And as you'll see from the following tips, some of these "smart" foods are also some of the tastiest.

1. Order up a spinach omelette for your eyes. According to a University of Texas Medical School study, egg yolks and spinach are good sources of lutein and zeaxanthin, phytochemicals that may help prevent age-related macular degeneration, one of the leading causes of blindness.

2. Visit the local seafood shack for stroke prevention. Just one crab leg gives you 84 milligrams of magnesium and 351 milligrams of potassium. So what, you say? In a study published in the medical journal *Circulation*, researchers evaluated the diets of more than 40,000 men and found that those who ate foods high in these minerals had a 38 percent lower risk of having a stroke.

3. Cut cholesterol with corn on the cob. The cholesterol-lowering powers of oat bran are undeniable, but so, unfortunately, is its bland taste. Here's a better option: corn on the cob. Researchers have shown that when men on a low-fat diet ate corn bran, their LDL cholesterol (the bad stuff) levels dropped. "Corn bran contains high levels of hemicellulose, a fiber that produces a fatty acid that seems to be responsible for unclogging arteries," says Paul Walker, Ph.D., a nutrition researcher at Illinois State University in Normal. "Whole corn should have a similar effect."

4. If you don't like corn, go nuts. Recent review studies from Loma Linda University in California showed that incorporating almonds and walnuts into your diet can lead to an 8 to 12 percent reduction in LDL cholesterol. Other studies have associated eating nuts with a 30 to 50 percent reduction in the risk of coronary heart disease. If you want some variety, try pistachios. Researchers at the UCLA School of Medicine recently found that people who took in 20 percent of their calories from pistachios increased their levels of HDL cholesterol by 11 percent.

5. Chill for 20 minutes to lose the fat. The next time you have a craving for a thick pork chop or a juicy New York strip, trim away the outer rim of fat before slapping it on the grill. It's easier to trim the fat if you first pop the meat in the freezer for 20 minutes. Chilling also causes hidden fat to turn white, making it easier to spot and lop off.

6. **Have a glass of fortified OJ for your head and heart.** Orange juice contains folic acid, a vitamin that appears to lower the homocysteine level in your blood. That's important because high homocysteine levels have been associated with an increased risk of heart disease. And according to a study published in the *Journal of Nutrition*, increasing your intake of folic acid helps raise your level of choline—an essential nutrient that may help improve memory.

7. **Protect your prostate with a pumped-up sauce.** Lycopene may lower your risk of prostate cancer by as much as 35 percent. One of the best ways to slip it into your diet: Make spaghetti sauce with sliced carrots or yellow peppers. Not only do cooked tomato products contain the highest levels of lycopene, but adding foods rich in beta-carotene will guide the lycopene to your prostate gland. USDA researchers found that when men were simultaneously given beta-carotene and lycopene supplements, more lycopene ended up in their bodies. And eating spaghetti is a lot more fun than eating pills.

8. **Eat pork chops for additional prostate protection.** Lean chops are low in fat—only 6 grams each for loin cuts—and high in selenium. Two 3-ounce chops contain more than 88 micrograms of selenium—almost half the amount needed to reduce the risk of prostate cancer by 63 percent, according to a University of Arizona study.

9. **Score health benefits with bottled green tea.** Green tea is the handyman of health foods. It does a job on arthritis, antibiotic-resistant bacteria, and prostate-cancer cells. To get the 4 cups a day some researchers believe you need, drink your green tea cold and bottled. Lester Mitscher, Ph.D., a medicinal biochemist at the University of Kansas in Lawrence, analyzed several different bottled teas and found that Lipton's Green Tea and Passion Fruit and Snapple Green Tea with Lemon have nearly the same antioxidant levels as the freshly brewed variety.

10. **Serve up spaghetti and meatballs for Father's Day.** If you've tried everything and still can't turn a half hour of passion into 9 months of pregnancy, try eating spaghetti and meatballs. Whole-wheat pasta and red meat are both packed with zinc, which increases sperm production, and the tomato sauce is a good source of vitamin C. "Men who don't take in enough vitamin C have lower-quality sperm," explains Althea Zanecosky, R.D., a spokeswoman for the American Dietetic Association.

11. **Drink a beer a day to keep the stones away.** Approximately four out of five kidney-stone sufferers are men. Good thing we like beer. According to a study published in the *American Journal of Epidemiology*, Finnish researchers evaluated the eating habits of about 27,000 men and found that drinking one beer a day was associated with a 40 percent lower risk of developing kidney stones. One explanation: The hops in beer help to keep calcium from leaching out of bones and taking up residence in your kidneys.

12. **Cook up a pot of health-fortifying chili.** If you want all the health benefits of soy in downright delectable form, try cooking some chili. Make your next batch with lean ground beef and canned soybeans. Soybeans are a good source of isoflavones, phytochemicals that may lower your LDL-cholesterol level by as much as 13 percent and help inhibit the growth of prostate-cancer cells.

13. **Fight cancer with fish.** You probably have already heard that eating salmon helps prevent heart disease. Now there's another reason to scarf up salmon: It may also protect you from cancer. According to a study published in the *American Journal of Clinical Nutrition*, people who consumed two or more servings of fish per week had between 50 percent and 60 percent lower rates of stomach, colon, and pancreatic cancers. The researchers speculate that the fatty acids in fish such as salmon and tuna inhibit the growth of cancer cells.

14. **Soak, then smoke, for added flavor.** To add interesting flavors to grilled food, use wood chips on top of the charcoal. Soak the chips in water, beer, or wine for 20 minutes first. Try using apple, cherry, or maple chips for chicken, suggests Steven Raichlen, author of *The Barbecue Bible*. He recommends mesquite or pecan for beef; alder for salmon or turkey; oak for seafood; and hickory for pork. Use poker chips for your in-laws.

15. **Fight heart disease with oil and vinegar.** Salads are healthy. Salad dressings aren't. Break the stalemate by drizzling some canola oil and red-wine vinegar over your roughage. Like the vino you drink straight, red-wine vinegar contains flavonoids, which help keep your arteries clear by preventing platelets from clumping together. Canola oil contains monounsaturated fats that lower "bad" (LDL) cholesterol without affecting "good" (HDL) cholesterol levels.

16. **After a night in the wild, make like a monkey.** Second only to aspirin, bananas should be considered your best friends after a binge. They're easy for an unsteady stomach to digest, and they contain the B vitamins that were sapped out of your body by excessive alcohol consumption. Restoring your supply is important because you need B vitamins to think clearly. Bananas are also high in fructose, which will help speed the metabolism of alcohol and shorten your hangover.

17. **For a healthier dip, blend some beans.** Drain some canned white beans and puree them in a blender with lemon juice, some garlic, some white wine, Worcestershire sauce, and Dijon mustard. Presto! You've got yourself a great, fiber-rich bread spread or dip, says Susan Massaron, food specialist and director of the cooking school at the Pritikin Longevity Center in Santa Monica, California.

18. **Calm down with carbs.** If stress is getting the best of your nerves, think carbohydrate. Eating foods high in carbohydrates makes our brains produce the calming chemical serotonin. To take advantage of this effect, find a quiet place and have a low-fat carbohydrate snack. Snacks that involve crunching or sucking are especially soothing. Think popcorn, rice cakes, cereal, lollipops, frozen pops, and sour balls.

You can even precalm yourself. If you're about to go into a grueling meeting, treat yourself to some carbohydrates about a half-hour before, says Judith Wurtman, Ph.D., a nutrition research scientist at Massachusetts Institute of Technology in Cambridge. You'll need about 1½ ounces of carbohydrates—2 cups of Cheerios, for example—for the calming effect to take place, Dr. Wurtman says.

3

SEX

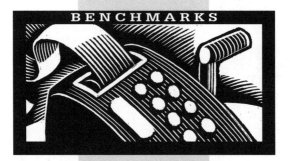

BENCHMARKS

■ Countries where women are twice as likely as American women to expect sex during the first week of dating: France, Italy, and Russia

■ The average number of times a year a man has sex: 79, or 1.5 times a week

■ The average number of sex partners a man has throughout his life: 12.4

■ The average number of sex partners a woman has throughout her life: 4

■ The average number of minutes a man lasts during sex: 14

■ The average number of minutes longer an uncircumcised man lasts: 4

■ The average number of seconds a man with premature ejaculation lasts: 24

■ The average number of times a man masturbates in a 1-week period: 1

■ The average number of times a man's risk of developing erectile problems increases after age 50: 3

■ The average number of sperm in a milliliter of semen: 100 million

■ The number of sperm in a milliliter of semen at which a man is considered infertile: 20 million

■ Percentage by which women are more likely to achieve multiple orgasms with uncircumcised men: 40

■ Percentage of sexual addicts who attempt suicide: 17

■ Ratio of husbands who say they fell in love with their spouses at first sight to wives who say this: 2:1

■ Percentage of newlyweds who say they had sex on the first date: 17

■ Years in jail for sex out of wedlock in Malaysia: 3

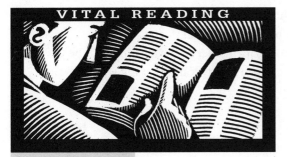

Common Causes of Equipment Failure

If last night wasn't the performance of a lifetime, learn what could be getting in your way.

Your penis isn't an Electrolux. Most things—vacuum cleaners, interns, your elbow—either work or they don't. But erections are a lot more complicated. A penis can be in perfect working condition and still refuse to stand and deliver. Take Colin, who at age 19 experienced a meltdown with one of the most beautiful women he knew. "It faded as I was putting the condom on. And it didn't return until after she'd left . . . disappointed."

Millions of guys can relate. "At some point in his life, every man fails to get an erection when he wants to," says Bill Finger, Ph.D., a psychologist at the VA Medical Center in Johnson City, Tennessee. If you haven't experienced unwanted downtime, it's only because your number hasn't been called yet. In most cases, nothing is wrong with the offending organ. Urologists estimate that in 80 percent of cases in men under 50, impotence isn't biological. It's what experts term situational impotence—a single incident brought on by external, not internal, factors. To prevent it from becoming more than a one-time thing, you need to understand what caused the problem in the first place.

Alcohol

We'd like to think we're better in the sack after our second longneck. But three's where we draw the line. According to a study conducted at Southern Illinois University, drinking more than 1.5 milliliters of alcohol per kilogram of body weight (for a 150-pound guy, that's 3½ drinks) caused drops in every measure of arousal the researchers looked at. Alcohol impairs your ability to harden the same way it impairs your ability to drive. Or walk. "It dulls the nerves that transmit sensation between your penis and your brain," says Laurence A. Levine,

M.D., an expert on male sexuality. Stay too long at the bar, loosening up for the night ahead, and your penis won't be able to walk.

Solution: If you're looking to perform later in the evening, tell the bartender to cut you off after three drinks. Beyond that, you're playing with firewater.

The Word "Impotence"

The watched kettle never boils, and the watched penis never hardens. "As long as you're focusing on getting hard, you're not giving yourself the chance to," says Dr. Finger. Any preoccupation with pelvic hydraulics replaces the erotic thoughts needed to make those hydraulics come to life.

Solution: When they suspect that an erection problem is temporary, some urologists attach an electronic device to the patient to record his overnight erections. "It's a great confidence booster, because when the results come back I can say, 'Wow, you were 90 percent rigid for 40 minutes last night—what a stud,'" says Dr. Finger.

You can get the same boost in confidence using no devices but your own. "If you have no problem with erections during masturbation, there's probably nothing physically wrong with you," Dr. Finger says.

The Past

If things didn't go well the last time you tried sex, this time is going to be even more difficult. "The more you replay the last time over and over in your head, the more likely you are to have problems," notes Dr. Finger.

Solution: Shift the blame. "If it happens just once and the man can't attribute it to something external and temporary, he assumes there's something wrong with him. But if you can find something to pin it on, you may be able to keep it from becoming a problem at all," says Dr. Finger. For example, perhaps it can be attributed to any of the following factors.

Your boss. Stress is one of an erection's biggest enemies, says Dr. Levine. And even if you're not consciously picturing coworkers or clients drifting over the headboard, the effect they've had on your body by the end of the day can take a while to wear off.

Solution: Change the scenery. "A change in setting is one of the first remedies I recommend for guys having performance problems, because it can help break the cycle of self-monitoring and performance anxiety," says Mark H. Cline, Ph.D., a psychologist in Dallas. Start with the guest bedroom or the backseat of that roomy new SUV. "Anything that breaks the routine is helpful," he says.

The troubled supermodel who thinks you're rich. For a guy prone to anxiety, a physically ideal partner can pose an even bigger problem than one with a few endearing flaws. "If a man is with a woman who's a 15 on a scale of 1 to 10, it can make him so anxious about his performance that he basically shuts down," says Dr. Levine.

Solution: Get to know her better first. Take more time during foreplay—investigate every nook and cranny. You'll become more comfortable, and your self-control will impress her. You hope.

The girl from Fotomat. Even if you haven't actually slept with her, any woman you've been fantasizing about can affect your ability to have erections when you're with your real partner. "I saw a guy a few months ago who became attracted to a woman, and even though they never had sex, he kissed her once and never told his wife about it. He felt so guilty that he developed an erection problem," says Dr. Finger. Affairs are so common among guys with erection problems that doctors routinely ask whether a patient is getting any on the side.

Solution: When you're alone, take your fantasy girl to bed. Screw her out of your system. (We're talking mentally, of course.) But keep the real sex between you and your partner. "There's nothing wrong with fantasizing about other women," says Dr. Finger. But don't act on these fantasies and don't tell your partner about them. Your honesty will not be appreciated.

Your position. Some positions are better than others for maintaining erections. "If you're on your back, it's possible to have what you can think of as a penis leak, where the blood actually flows out of your penis rather than staying in and keeping you hard," says Stacy Elliott, M.D., clinical associate professor at the University of British Columbia in Vancouver. Any position that causes your penis to bend in an unusual or painful way can also interfere with erections by replacing a pleasurable, erection-friendly sensation with a painful, erection-dampening one.

Solution: Stick to the missionary position. "If you're on top, gravity's helping blood to pool in your penis," says Dr. Elliott.

Your drug habit. Dozens of prescription drugs list erection problems as a side effect, most commonly antidepressants, blood-pressure drugs, prostate shrinkers, diuretics, and antiulcer drugs. But don't trust your doctor to warn you. "Some doctors feel it's better not to suggest that a drug might cause erection problems, especially for a guy who's already having anxiety about his performance," explains Dr. Finger.

Solution: Make sure your doctor knows that erections are a priority for you, and ask that he prescribe only drugs that won't interfere. And don't assume that a drug is safe just because it's sold over the counter. Antihistamines (found in cold remedies), naproxen (found in Aleve), ibuprofen (found in Advil and Motrin), and some sleeping pills can interfere with erections.

Too much masturbation. We have nothing against practicing for the main event. In fact, frequent erections and regular ejaculation help keep your sexual parts primed. But sometimes athletes who overtrain end up losing the race. The danger: You'll be so accustomed to getting it exactly the way you like it that any woman who tries to please you will end up failing.

Solution: Cut back on the amount of time you spend attending to personal business, and when you do masturbate, focus on techniques that mimic intercourse. Thrust against a loosely cuffed hand rather than pumping with your fist, for example. Also, ask your partner to work more manual and oral stimulation into foreplay to help keep your erection hard until penetration.

The Truth behind the Measurements

Here's how to take advantage of what you've been given.

Having sex is no great achievement. Insert Tab A into Slot B, and there you have it. Good sex, however, is a little more complicated and a hell of a lot more fun. To achieve that, you first have to take a look at what you're bringing to the party. Really, take a look at it. Is it long? Short? Wide? False modesty or, worse, comparing yourself to the lumber at Home Depot isn't helpful. You need to be objective, which means you'll need to measure.

Before you balk at the idea of locking yourself in the bathroom with a ruler, consider this: Spend just 5 minutes calculating the length, girth, and erection angle of your penis, and you can spend the rest of your life having better sex. Once you know your dimensions, we'll show you ways to use what you have more effectively.

Sizing Yourself Up

Most men go through life without a clear idea of how big they actually are. In fact, researchers have found that the average man thinks he's below average.

"Men were good at appraising their overall physique, but when it came to relative penis size, as a group they tended to underestimate," says Peter A. Lee, M.D., of the University of Pittsburgh. Twenty-six percent of respondents to Dr. Lee's study gauged their own penis size as "below average," but a mere 5 percent checked the "above average" box.

"It's difficult to accurately assess penis size," Dr. Lee says. The damn thing is always getting bigger or smaller, and your point of view can be misleading. "If you're in a locker room with other men, theirs may look bigger because you're seeing them in profile. You look down at your own."

The best way to tell how big you are is to measure yourself as a urologist would. We asked the University of Arizona's Hunter Wessells, M.D., who has studied penis size, to tell us how. You can compare your answers with the averages below, compiled from recent studies in the United States and Australia.

- Flaccid length: Measure immediately after undressing, since a cold or warm room can cause shrinkage or expansion. Do it while standing, and use a flexible ruler. "Position the tip of the ruler gently against the point where the shaft meets the abdomen," says Dr. Wessells. Then simply bend the ruler along the shaft and read the length. Average: 3.43 inches.
- Erect length: Immediately after you become fully hard, measure along the top of your erection from the base of the shaft to the tip. Average: 5.03 inches.
- Girth: While still erect, wrap a cloth tape measure around your penis at its base. Average: 5.14 inches around; 1.67 inches in diameter.
- Erection angle: Stand with your back against a wall and estimate your angle. A zero-degree erection (an oxymoron if we've ever heard one) would point at your feet; 90 degrees would point directly out in front; and 180 degrees would point up at your chin. Average: 105.7 degrees.

Make the Most of What You Have

Now that you know what you're working with, it's time to learn how to use it to your best advantage.

If your erect length is:

6.5 inches or more: Though you probably feel that you have the advantage over every other guy, your partner may not agree. "I hear many more horror stories from women about large penises than I hear crying over small ones," says Bernie Zilbergeld, Ph.D., a sex therapist. That's because having the back of the vagina struck during intercourse is painful for many women, generating the same nauseated feeling you get when you bump a testicle. So with length comes responsibility. Don't thrust too deeply when you're on top. Or else lie back and let your partner straddle you with her knees on the bed. When she wants to use the top of your penis, she'll keep her knees close to your body and thrust gently against the tip of your erection. If she wants more, she'll slide her knees outward and lower herself as far as is comfortable.

4.5 to 6.4 inches: Most of the vagina's nerves are located in its outer third, the area you're best equipped to delight. "The man who learns how to tease a woman at the outset—by putting it partway in and taking it out—will be perceived as a better lover than the guy who uses his full length to drill for gold," says Mark L. Elliott, Ph.D., director of the Institute for Psychological and Sexual Health.

An average-size man can better target this sensitive outer third by entering from on top while the woman lies with her legs flat on the bed. This reduces the depth of penetration by preventing your pelvises from coming all the way together. (This is also a good position for oversize guys.) In addition, when her legs are extended, it puts more tension on her vaginal lips, which improves the stimulation for both of you.

Less than 4.5 inches: "Men who are short sometimes feel cheated, but they have options that larger men don't have," says Judy Seifer, Ph.D., a sex therapist.

When a woman first becomes aroused, her vagina expands more than necessary to accommodate an object it hasn't yet had a chance to size up. "Then, after a minute or two of thrusting, it collapses back around the penis," says Dr. Elliott.

Use this to your advantage by employing the coital alignment technique. "You simply ride high, bringing the base of your penis up against her clitoris," says Dr. Seifer. Then, instead of thrusting, rub and grind against her pubic bone. "Since you're not thrusting, it doesn't matter how long or short you are; it's all in the rocking motion."

If you're worried about your appearance with the lights on, try trimming your pubic hair. "A careful trim will make you look an inch and a half longer," notes Dr. Seifer. Snip half an inch or so around the base of your penis. Don't do this after drinking.

If your girth is:

More than 5.14 inches: A guy with a thick penis and a girl with a small vagina can make for an unhappy couple. "I've actually heard of a few cases where there were such dramatic size differences that it was just too painful for the woman to have sex," says Dr. Elliott. Although that's rare, men in this category need to exercise caution, especially during the transition from foreplay to intercourse.

Keep in mind that the more aroused your partner becomes during foreplay, the more her vagina will expand. "So simply waiting for her to get wet isn't good enough," Dr. Elliott cautions. "You have to wait several minutes more, until she's fully engorged. She'll eventually accommodate you." Then use a little saliva or lube to moisten your penis before entry. Ask her to guide you in, and go easy on the first dozen thrusts.

5.14 inches or less: For men with narrow penises, it's all about friction. "Women don't usually have a problem with thin guys, but some men say they can't achieve enough sensation and they feel like they're lost inside the vagina," says Dr. Seifer. If this has been your experience, the best position for lovemaking is one in which the woman's knees are together and her vagina is stretched from front to back, not side to side. She can either lie flat on the bed or tuck her legs up against her chest. This will pull her vaginal lips together, tightening her grip on your erection and creating extra friction.

A great position for a man with a long, thin penis is to enter from behind while she lies flat on her stomach. This reduces depth and increases tightness.

If your erection angle is:

90 degrees or more: The more directly skyward your penis points, the less flexible your erection is and the more careful you have to be when using it. It's possible to fracture your penis, so don't get too acrobatic during sex, and be especially careful when she's gyrating on top. Also, "note which way you point, and consider the angle of your partner's vagina," says Dr. Seifer. Take a finger, explore, and try to get a sense of which way she slants. "Deep upward thrusts can put uncomfortable pressure on the back wall of a woman's bladder, which can give her the urge to urinate." If your angle is steep, ask her to sit up against the headboard for better alignment.

If your erection curves slightly toward the ceiling (about 25 percent of erections do), you possess the perfect penis to rub her G-spot. Use the missionary position, but keep your pelvis low and make shallow thrusts. Steep, stubby men are doubly blessed: They can keep the head of the penis within those first sensitive inches of the vagina and stimulate the G-spot at the same time.

Less than 90 degrees: Don't be upset if you have a low angle of erection. Positions that don't work for others—such as face-to-face sex, where the two of you sit and then lie back connected only at the hips—can give you a creative advantage.

Find positions that give you maximum stimulation. For most men, this means the missionary position. "It helps keep the blood flow going, which increases sensitivity and endurance, and may help boost erection angle," says Elliott.

If you point or curve to the left or right, be extra careful during sex: A misaligned penis can be very uncomfortable for your partner, especially during the initial thrusts. "A lot of men with penises that point to 10 or 2 o'clock find that sideways positions such as spooning work best at first," says Dr. Seifer.

Multiple Orgasms

Check out these five easy steps to giving the sexual performance of your life.

When you try to cram multiple orgasms into one night, they often turn out like the Rocky movies: The first one is great, the second is about half as good, and you can forget about the third, fourth, and fifth.

It didn't always work this way. When you were 15, all it took was a Farrah poster and a locked door and you were set for the afternoon. Now that you're older, however, your body has changed. You need a break. Urologists call it the refractory period; that's the time it takes for your penis to go from one ejaculation to the next erection.

On most nights, you're probably satisfied with your typical output—one and done. But multiple erections do have their advantages. First, you'll impress and excite any woman, because you'll be the man who can last as long as she can. It's wedding-night sex, any night. You may also find that your erections the second and third time around are stronger and longer lasting. More pleasure for everyone.

So why stop at a single helping? Here's the plan for hitting the bedroom the way you hit the buffet line.

1. **Build up steam.** Before you even think about undressing her, you have to train your brain and body for the long night ahead. Make sure you follow these pre-bedroom tactics:

 • Keep your distance. Todd Shackelford, Ph.D., a psychologist at Florida Atlantic University in Boca Raton, found that men reported a 10 percent increase in their sexual desire for every 100 hours they spent apart from their partners. If you're planning a big night—an anniversary, for instance—limit the amount of time you spend with her for a couple of days beforehand.

 • Even if you're flying solo, keep your hands off the stick. To reduce your recovery time in bed, don't masturbate for several days before your date. "The more you ejaculate, the longer your refractory periods," explains Dudley Seth Danoff, M.D., urologic surgeon at Cedars-Sinai Medical Center in Los Angeles. Psychologically, the layoff increases your level of lust. Physiologically, the buildup guarantees a full tank when you need it.

 • Take her out for a fancy dinner. Make sure it's a place where she'll wear her sexiest stuff. If fellow diners spend more time staring at her strapless black dress than at their lobster tails, you're successfully greasing the wheel. "If a guy perceives his partner as sexually attractive to other men, that makes the guy more interested in sex with her," says Dr. Shackelford. And urologists agree that the higher your desire, the sturdier your penis.

2. **Skip the romance.** Now that she's naked, consider your first erection the sacrificial lamb. Too much stimulation early on can actually desensitize your penis later, so limit the foreplay for now and start thrusting as soon as it's practical. "Men with premature ejaculation often report that their second erections are longer lasting and thus better," says James Barada, M.D., a urologist and the director of the Center for Male Sexual Health in Albany, New York. Lather her up for a quickie, climax as fast as you can, and reassure her that this sudden quake is going to be followed by a devastating aftershock.

3. **Speed the recovery.** Before you can have another erection, the smooth muscles that constrict during orgasm need to relax completely. "That way, the cells in your penile tissue will rest long enough to be ready for your next erection," Dr. Barada says. To better your bounce-back time, follow these steps.

- Swap massages. Relieving tension in any of your muscles decreases anxiety, a factor in secondary erections. Massage her first. A tip: Stay away from your favorite areas of her body during the first part of the massage. You need rest, not more excitement.
- Ask her to get out of bed and bring back beer. Alcohol in low doses actually helps increase the arousal signals from your brain to your penile tissue, Dr. Barada says. Your inhibitions are down, so you're more easily excited than if you were completely sober (a lesson you should have learned at your first frat party). "But after two drinks, alcohol acts as a potent depressant. And though it may delay an orgasm, it decreases your ability to have another erection," Dr. Barada says.

  When you've downed your beer, get out of bed yourself and dispose of the empties. Good circulation is also important in maintaining strong erections, and you can improve your blood flow just by standing up and moving around.
- Skip any post-romp cigarettes. Nicotine kills erections faster than a rerun of *The Golden Girls*.

4. **Introduce party favors.** As if they needed a study to prove this: Korean researchers showed that, among 45 men, the rigidity of erections decreased by nearly 15 percent from the first time they watched an erotic video to the third time they watched the very same video. It's a simple fact: To stay hard, you need to change your stimuli.

For repeat performances, always treat every time as if it were the first time. You can do that simply by experimenting with different tactile sensations. Most people use oil or lotion, but you can do better, says Michael Seiler, Ph.D., a sex therapist and the director of the Phoenix Institute in Chicago. Raid your closet for two pairs of fur-lined gloves: one for you, one for her. Wear them inside out.

The new sensation of fur rubbing flesh should make you appreciate the joys of the wild kingdom.

5. **Let Nature do the work.** Until now, you've done all the heavy lifting. So by night's end, you deserve some help. A 35-year-old man has anywhere from two to eight involuntary erections during the night, says Jacques Susset, M.D., clinical professor of urology at Brown University in Providence, Rhode Island. Each one lasts anywhere from 10 minutes to an hour. So just before you doze off, set your alarm for 3 hours later. With any luck, your penis will be up before you. Spoon her to demonstrate your interest, and you're on for the third act. Take a bow afterward.

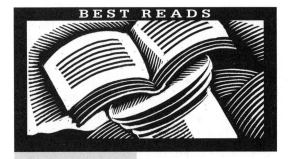

BEST READS

Set the Right Mood

When it comes to sex, most men hate anticipation. It gets in the way. But if you want to enjoy your time between the sheets tonight, you need to know that women love anticipation. For them, anticipation is the way. As authors Laurence Roy Stains and Stefan Bechtel point out in this excerpt from What Women Want *(Rodale), a day of phone calls and compliments and affection is all part of mental foreplay.*

You're about to hear some pure, out-and-out girl talk. At times, it will be so nicey-nice, so unfailingly polite, that it will make your teeth ache.

So we're going to cut you a break, right here up front. We're going to start with the translation into guy speak. Here's the take-home message, as translated for us by Jane, a 30-year-old mother of two in El Cajon, California:

> *If he's been an asshole all day and then he's only nice for 10 minutes, that doesn't do it.*

You have to set a mood.

This is not some minor detail that maybe you can overlook except on Valentine's Day. Let's put it this way. . . . You know how important foreplay is to women, right? Well, here's the point: They think that setting the mood is part of foreplay.

We are not kidding.

"Foreplay starts long before you hop into bed," says Lorri in Washington State.

Do you feel like a deer caught in the headlights?

"Foreplay begins way before the bedroom. If he's understanding and considerate during the day, sex is always better at night."

So says Connie in central Pennsylvania. The women we surveyed indicate that she speaks for women everywhere.

One Vancouver woman even calls it romantic foreplay.

And Laura, a 32-year-old Web site developer in New York City, refers to romance as "the mental side of foreplay."

To most guys, the very idea of mental foreplay is, like, out there. But to most women, the idea is right here. That's because, for us, the upward climb to orgasm is pretty much a matter of penile stimulation. But for them, it's not strictly a matter of genital arousal. They claim that the brain is their biggest sex organ. One of our intrepid in-depth interviewers went so far as to say, "Women are sexual from the brain on down; and men are sexual from the dick up."

Maria, a 24-year-old student in Chicago, puts it most simply. She said, "A big portion of good sex occurs in my head."

When you realize this fundamental difference between the sexes, a lot of things start to fall into place. As Karen in Hilliard, Florida, makes clear in this *New Woman* magazine survey response:

> *For most women, sex is between the ears. (In other words, what sets the flame, fans it, and creates the biggest infernos is what happens in the brain beforehand—words, innuendoes, looks, small touches, a single kiss, etcetera.) It's like a Christmas present: The longer you have to look at the wrapped package under the tree, the more wonderful the anticipation and the more you want to open it. Why do you think women love reading romance novels so much? Those books are 99 percent buildup, 1 percent action.*

The flip side of that is: no buildup, no action. Let's look at the specific components of a good buildup.

Touch her in a loving but no-strings-attached way. "Everyone likes being touched," says Wendy, a 26-year-old programmer in New York City. "I really like being touched. I remember one time my boyfriend brushed my hair for about half an hour and I was so wet—I just had orgasms for days. I was, like, crying afterward, and he was, like, 'What's wrong, honey?'"

For some women, it's especially arousing if you display your affection in public. "Public shows of affection make me feel proud and cared for," says Kathy in Peoria, Illinois.

Anna in Huntington Beach, California, agrees. "To me, the sexiest thing a man can do is to make me feel sexy when other people are around—to make me feel like we're the only two people there."

And here's a promise from an anonymous respondent to our survey: "Take more time to be romantic instead of, 'How about you and me go upstairs.' If there was hugging, touching, and kissing ahead of time, he wouldn't have to ask to go upstairs. It would happen where we were."

Be an old-fashioned chauvinist—her chauvinist. You know, this stuff worked for eons, and Angela in California is one of many women who think it still works. "Opening the door for you, taking your arm as you walk, anything like that," she says. "There aren't a lot of men who do that anymore."

Pay her a compliment. "I wish he would be more complimentary about my body," says Catherine in Chicago, of her boyfriend. "He isn't. And it shuts me down a little bit. For the most part, I am happy about the way I look, but it would be nice to get some feedback about that. I think he feels a little bit burdened about my insecurity around it."

Laura in New York City really lays it on the line: "The less I hear it, the less I think of myself physically. And if I don't feel attractive around him, I'm not going to want to have sex. If I don't feel like I'm beautiful then, you know, I'm going to be a lot more intimidated when I take my clothes off, when I start to do things to his body. I'm going to feel a lot more insecure. I think more men really need to understand that they have to kiss up, I guess."

Compliments are critically important to women who are not a pert, perky size four anymore. If she has any weight problems or beauty issues or body-image issues, she'll need you to be expressive. Eunice in Louisiana wrote to say, "Lately, I've been feeling self-conscious about my weight. This caused me to have a decreased sexual drive for awhile. When I spoke about it, my husband was encouraging. He said he found me to be sexy and likened my body to the women in the famous Renaissance paintings and sculptures. Our sex life became almost immediately better. I still need to watch my weight, but at the same time I feel desirable."

Other women don't want compliments about appearances. For instance, Alice, a 46-year-old nurse in Canada, says, "I love a compliment about something

I've done. I'm more of a concrete person in that respect. A good dinner that I've worked hard on . . . I love compliments like that, where he's giving me credit. That sets me up. I'm really easy then."

Pardon the shouting, but the overall point is to *make her feel appreciated.* Mandy in Pennsylvania puts it nicely: "Don't we all feel a little bit more adventuresome when we feel good about ourselves? We really feel like glory."

As a final thought: Timing is everything. Don't wait until you're in bed to pay a compliment, or your sincerity will be suspect. She'll assume it's your dumb stick talking. One woman gave us this advice: "Never tell a woman she's beautiful when the lights are off."

Pay attention. Talk to her. When men talk, they share information. When women talk, they share feelings. The act of talking, in itself, is intimate. Maybe that explains why a woman in Waterbury, Connecticut, wrote, "Good foreplay for me is hours of conversation over a really good bottle of wine."

Denise in Massachusetts feels the same. "A guaranteed way to turn me on would be having a completely open, honest, intimate conversation. Being uninhibited with my partner makes me feel real connected to my partner. When the conversation is followed by lots of kissing, stroking, cuddling, and touching, I am totally turned on and ready for a night of wild, hot, passionate sex."

We could continue to quote women saying stuff like, "Foreplay is an all-day, all-night event." Clearly, some women could talk about it all day and all night. Here's the topper: Andrea in Ohio saying, "Foreplay is maybe a way of life." This is where most men get lost, because these women have gotten a little too dreamy—their scenarios sound like a daytime soap opera.

But you should see their real lives. Kate in Chicago gives us a glimpse of her reality when she says, "Sitting around, drinking beer, and watching television for a couple of hours makes me not that interested in having sex."

Kate likes to get out in the evenings. But if you do stay home, well, that doesn't have to be all bad. It's what you make of it. Compare Kate's home life to this scene:

"Foreplay is anything that happens before sex that is sensual," says Sarah Jane, a 43-year-old consultant in Michigan. "I mean, I have had dinner where we made pasta puttanesca, and I wore my bra and put a linen napkin in it. He wore his underwear. We had a blast. That, to me, is foreplay."

When the mood builds, don't blow it. We may be making this setting-the-mood thing sound like more of a burden than it has to be. You know, most women are like Kate—all you really have to do is go out for a great night with them, and the mood is set automatically. In that case, your only job is not screwing up once you get back home.

Lori, a 28-year-old computer consultant in Fort Lee, New Jersey, makes an excellent point:

> *I have this thing that, whenever we get dressed up and go out for a night on the town, if I'm wearing a skirt and heels, that means it's supposed to be a romantic night. A sexual night because we're dressed up. Those are missed opportunities, otherwise, because I'm always feeling prettier when I'm in a sexy dress. So the trick is, when we first walk back in the door, to keep my mood going and kiss me or throw me against the wall, or pick me up and throw me into bed.*
>
> *But don't wait for me to brush my teeth and take off my dress and get in my pajamas, because by then it's missed. Don't turn on the lights and check for messages and get on the phone. Don't come home and start talking about the scores of the baseball game. This is not the night for it.*

And now that you're both mentally ready for bed, what do you do to get ready physically? We put this question to our 80 in-depth interview subjects: "A lot of men love it when a woman wears lingerie to bed. But what can a man do before he comes to bed?"

The overwhelming, nearly universal reply was "Take a shower."

Remember, "Women," as one said, "are olfactory people." Perhaps you hadn't noticed, but their sense of smell is keener than yours. It's not just that they want you not to smell bad. Women think a freshly showered man smells good. Sexy, even.

"I think it's awesome if a man comes to bed and smells like soap," says Catherine, a 24-year-old Canadian studying in the Midwest.

The runner-up reply was "Brush your teeth."

"It's all in the breath. He needs to brush his teeth, or I can't do it," says Kate, a Chicago attorney.

"It's amazing how many times a man will get into bed and not realize that his pizza-and-beer breath is a turn-off," says Anna from Huntington Beach, California.

We think this is pretty good news, actually. After the demanding tone of the requests for more romantic foreplay, this is refreshing. Women aren't expecting that much of us at bedtime. A bar of soap, a bottle of mouthwash, and thou. That's it. Oh, and if it's your place, not hers: clean sheets. Can you handle that? For women, love is a front-end operation.

So light a few candles. Put on some music. No, there's no secret sex music that will drive her wild. Most of our 80 interviewees like music in the background during lovemaking, but their tastes run the gamut from rock to reggae to classical. It's not like they all said, "Oh, I'll go down on anyone who plays the Cranberries."

But here's one tip: Now is perhaps the time to play that CD of hers that you really hate. You know, one of those Lilith Fair female vocalists. You may get a reaction. "One of my favorite experiences was Fiona Apple—'Criminal,'" recalls Danielle from Philadelphia. "That song . . . it's a very female empowering song, and I just crawled all over him and completely took control."

What about underwear? Is there the male equivalent of a Victoria's Secret scarlet teddy? Not really. Our in-depth interviewees preferred silk boxers over briefs. But they gagged at the thought of you wearing something that you think might be sexy. "Men turn me on," says Wendy, "but I don't want to look at them in a rubber G-string or anything."

Susi, a Philadelphia mother of two, recalls, "I had a boyfriend once who wore bikini underwear to bed. I was, like, 'Go join the Chippendales.' I thought it was so stupid."

Chances are, the underwear you should wear is already tucked away in your dresser drawer. It's the underwear that she gave you, doofus. "I like it when he just wears his cute little boxers that I buy for him," says Carly, a New York City teacher.

The women we grilled were largely indifferent to cologne. They don't care whether Fido or Snowball is in the room. Whether the lights are on or off is strictly a matter of personal preference. (A 29-year-old Alabama woman tells us, "Bright overhead light makes me feel like I'm at the gynecologist's office.")

And although some women think it's erotic if you leave one item of clothing on, most do not. Mostly, they want you to take off your socks. "The socks have got to come off," says Catherine. "Unless it's a quickie, where he's still wearing his pants and you can't see the whole leg/sock ratio. But if he's totally naked except for one piece of clothing, that's ridiculous."

"Get those stupid socks off," says Kristen, a 29-year-old teacher in Chicago. "The last thing we want to see is a guy walking around half-naked with socks on."

"Yes! Yes!" agrees Dawn, a 21-year-old student in Maine. "One time, he left his shoes on. Oh, God!"

Take the Monotony Out of Monogamy

Has your sex life become like the summer reruns? Same time, same place, same plot? Fortunately, marriage doesn't have to equal monotony—not when there are so many ways to liven things up. In this excerpt from Good Loving *(Rodale), authors Donna Raskin, Larry Keller, and the editors of* Men's Health *Books share some candid advice about ways to rekindle the sparks in your relationship—both in and out of the bedroom.*

There is no reason to be sexually bored in a monogamous relationship. No reason, that is, except for a few million years of polygamous human evolution. And a brain constructed without any consideration for monogamy. And a natural human preference for sexual novelty and variety. And some subtle "permission" from society to fool around. And all the attendant pressures of just being in the same house with the same person every day.

Come to think of it, we should rephrase the question. Is there any reason *not* to be sexually bored in a monogamous relationship?

Yes, and it's worth it. The monotony monster is eminently slayable. The secret is the oldest battle strategy known to man: Know thy enemy, and you can whip it. In this case, your opponent is called biology.

The basic problem is simple. "You're fighting a genuine restlessness born from millennia of having sexual variety being part of basic human reproductive strategy," says Helen Fisher, Ph.D., research associate in the department of anthropology at Rutgers University in New Brunswick, New Jersey, and author of *Anatomy of Love*. "I don't think the human animal was built to be with one person for the rest of his life," she says. "So the sexual boredom that can set in with monogamy is real."

It's not that we're evil or sinful or unable to make commitments, says Robert Birch, Ph.D., a psychologist in Columbus, Ohio, who specializes in marriage and sex therapy and is author of *Male Sexual Endurance*. "It's just that we're struggling with our biology." Sex researchers agree that there's something about us that equates novelty with excitement. At the same time, the very definition of monogamy makes novelty impossible. Houston, we've got a problem.

Nurturing Novelty

"If novelty weren't sexually exciting, how would Hugh Hefner have created his empire?" Dr. Birch says. Good point. One centerfold serves its purpose as well as any other, but it was the appearance of a new one every month that built the Playboy mansion.

And, let's face it, in the novelty competition, monogamy struggles to keep up. "Marital sex won't be as 'exciting' as an affair," says Dr. Birch. "A long-term relationship doesn't have the novelty, the risk, the danger, and the forbidden aspects of an affair. That's just reality."

But it's also reality that we don't live in nature. We may be animals, but we're not *animals*. We want monogamy; we just don't want it to be dull. Our evolutionary heritage is a challenge, not a sentence. If shortcomings in the novelty department are the problem with monogamy, there are ways to fight it. A good start: Take the monotony out of monogamy by putting novelty in, starting with these suggestions.

Bust the rut. Same time, same place, same way, every time. You're on the fast track to booorrrring. Routine guarantees monotony. But couples fall into routines as easily as they fell in love. And then they wonder why they're bored. "You have to do something to make it different and exciting," says Isadora Alman, a San Francisco sexologist who writes the syndicated sex and relationship advice column "Ask Isadora." She adds, "Even the most incredible lover imaginable has to be more than a one-trick pony."

So instead of poking this and rubbing that every Wednesday night during Letterman, try poking and rubbing on a Tuesday night during Leno. Throw in a lick here or a nuzzle there while you're at it. Hey, it's a start.

Put sex in prime time. Rut happens. And time management is often the culprit. You have your work, she has hers; you both have the kids. Sex gets relegated to the back burner or gets taken off the stove entirely. That's boring. Rearrange your priorities, says Timothy Perper, Ph.D., a Philadelphia biologist, independent sex researcher, and author of *Sex Signals: The Biology of Love.* "It's a ghastly cliché," he says, "but you have to set aside quality time for your sex life together."

And to qualify as "quality," this time has to be at least as prime (though maybe not as long) as what you give to your work, and, yes, to your kids. After midnight on exhausting days doesn't cut it. "How can you enjoy sex when you're in no condition to enjoy anything?" asks sex therapist Theresa Crenshaw, M.D., author of *The Alchemy of Love and Lust.* "You can't operate on burnout and expect sex to function."

Make it a project. Pay as much attention to your sexual relationship as you do to your work (or sports, or your car), and you'll fend off boredom, says Dr. Fisher. Approach it like a project. That means doing the research (books, tapes, videos), exploring the possibilities, identifying your needs, testing alternatives, practicing the technical tricks. In other words, everything you do when you buy a computer or join a fantasy baseball league.

"There are all kinds of ways to combat boredom, but you have to make the effort," Dr. Fisher says. "Too many men get caught like a mouse on a treadmill. They complain about how boring it is—but they never get off the wheel."

Don't *work* at your relationship. Yes, you read that right. True, you do have to make the effort to keep the zing in your sex life. But if you think of it as work, you're losing the battle. In fact, that's a big reason why some couples throw in the towel, says Barry McCarthy, Ph.D., a Washington, D.C., psychologist for the Washington Psychological Center and author of *Male Sexual Awareness.* "When couples stop having sex, it's almost always the man's call," he says. "He figures if it's going to be more of a hassle than a pleasure, then it's not worth it." So don't hassle. Enjoy the process. Think of Operation Anti-Monotony as an exploration, an adventure. "Sustaining the sexual chemistry isn't work," says Dr. Crenshaw. "It wasn't work when you were doing all those things to orchestrate special evenings with your conquest of the week. Keep that sense of pleasure."

Assume she'll cooperate. Don't short-circuit your anti-monotony efforts out of fear that she may not be in the spirit of things. Remember, she doesn't like ennui any more than you. And if you're bored, odds are she is, too. "People don't get bored by themselves; relationships get boring," Dr. Fisher says. "If you come up with a good idea, she'll probably go for it."

Hang in there. As you make that broken-field run toward sexual pay dirt within your relationship, you're going to have to dodge some temptations to give up. "You have all kinds of things set up for you to escape," says Kathleen Gill, Ph.D., a clinical psychologist, certified sex therapist, and adjunct professor of psychology at Harvard Medical School. "You have access to pornography, prostitutes, cybersex, affairs." The point, says Dr. Gill, isn't that these things are evil, but rather that our culture, by winking at transgressions by men, makes it easy to lose track of the larger goal.

Injecting novelty into your sex play is a useful ongoing pick-me-up, a proven boredom-killer. But you need to make a more fundamental change in your approach to sex if you want to weed out monotony at its roots.

How? Dr. McCarthy calls the answer interactive sex. It comes down to intimacy, to exploiting the arousal inherent in you, in her, and in the interaction between you. "If you buy only the notion that what makes sex hot is a new stimulant from the outside, you wind up devaluing ongoing sex and de-eroticizing your partner," Dr. McCarthy says. "It's as if you don't own your own sexuality, that it's something external to you." So take responsibility for your own arousal instead of wondering why it doesn't "happen." Stop chasing lightning and build a fire instead.

Getting Intimate—Again

Sexual boredom is sometimes nothing more than a cave-in to intimacy overload, says Louanne Cole Weston, Ph.D., a board-certified sex therapist; a marriage, family, and child counselor; and a sex columnist for the *San Francisco Examiner*. "When you feel you're getting overloaded with all the intimacy that accumulates in a relationship, sex is the place where you turn it down," Dr. Weston says. "Sex is the one thing that's optional. Raising the kids or putting food on the table isn't."

Here are some ways to blast boredom and restore intimacy to your love life.

Get together. Connecting sexually is easier if it's just one more aspect of other kinds of intimacy. In case you haven't noticed, men and women are pretty busy these days, so it's important to set aside time to be together somewhere outside the bedroom. Alman calls it sweetheart time, but just pretend you never heard the term. The important thing is to do it. "It doesn't necessarily have to be time for sex," Alman says. "But if you build in sweetheart time, sex follows."

Share an adventure. While a woman's idea of intimacy is talking, a man's is doing. So try to get her to do things with you that tap your sense of intimacy. "Men love adventure," Dr. Fisher says. "A side-by-side adventure is intimacy for a man, just as it was on the grasslands of Africa a million years ago."

Try a long walk in the city with no set destination. Your prey? The unknown bookstore, the hidden park, the street you didn't know was there.

Soak her in. Okay, you've had your adventure together. Now try it her way. That means talk. "You have to recognize that face-to-face talking is intimacy to her," Dr. Fisher says. Find a conversation-conducive setting that holds out some other attractions and approach it in good faith. Try talking in the tub, for example.

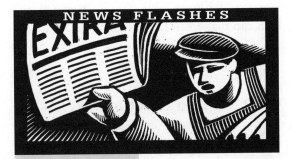

NEWS FLASHES

Sex after Prostate Surgery Possible with New Procedure

HOUSTON—Surgeons may be able to prevent impotence in men having their prostates removed. During a radical prostatectomy, a surgeon can simply remove a small ankle nerve and graft it onto erection-producing nerves that may have been damaged or severed. Sixty men have received the graft, and many are gradually regaining their sexual function. "Four of the first 12 men, who would normally have no chance of having a viable erection again, were able to have intercourse a year after the procedure," says Edward Kim, M.D., a urologist at Baylor College of Medicine in Houston. Ask your urologist if this procedure is available in your area.

Antidepressant Could Delay Ejaculation

SYDNEY, Australia—A few years ago, men taking antidepressants such as Anafranil and Prozac discovered that they didn't ejaculate as quickly. So physicians began prescribing daily doses to men suffering from premature ejaculation. That caused other side effects; some men even temporarily lost their ability to ejaculate at all. But Australian researchers have discovered that you can delay ejaculation by taking an antidepressant right before sex—you needn't take it every day. In a study at St. Luke's Hospital Complex in Sydney, 26 men began taking 20 milligrams of Paxil 4 hours before having sex, and their time to ejaculation increased from just 18 seconds to more than 3 minutes. Ask your doctor for more details.

Frequent Sex May Make You Look Younger

EDINBURGH, Scotland—Sex just may be one of the best antiaging remedies around. During an 18-year study, David Weeks, Ph.D., a Scottish researcher, interviewed 3,500 people about their sex lives. When a panel of researchers tried to guess the subjects' ages, they thought the men who had sex three or more times a week looked an average of 12 years younger than they actually were. "Having sex helps the body produce growth hormones that produce lean muscle tissue and decrease body fat, which can make you look younger," explains Dr. Weeks. It's hardly hard science, but it's nice to think sex can keep your face smooth.

Researchers Discover New Factor in Erection Strength

ROME, Italy—Men might think they need only one thing in order to have an erection: a penis. In fact, a new Italian study shows that the strength of the muscles surrounding the penis may also play a part. When researchers studied the strength of two pelvic-area muscles in 390 men, they found that potent guys were 17 percent stronger than the guys who had trouble with erections. "These muscles squeeze the two blood-filled erection tubes in the penis. The stronger these muscles are, the more pressure they'll create in the erection," says Gregory A. Broderick, M.D., a Mayo Clinic urologist. By simply squeezing and releasing the muscles you use to stop urination, you can train these muscles to get stronger.

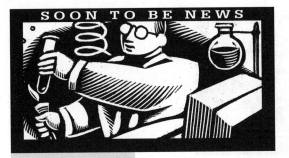

SOON TO BE NEWS

Hormone Injection More Effective Than the Pill?

About 5 percent of women who take the Pill get pregnant, but a new female contraceptive may be able to improve those odds. In a 15-month University of Florida study of 1,103 women, none of the 782 women who received a monthly hormone injection called Lunelle became pregnant; two of the 321 women on the Pill did. "This is a level of effectiveness you'd expect from sterilization," says Andrew Kaunitz, M.D., the lead investigator.

The injection should be widely available soon.

A South American Sex Enhancer?

Maca is a plant native to Peru that has a reputation as a libido lifter. When scientists from PureWorld Botanicals fed maca extracts to male mice, they got some surprising results. The maca-free mice had sex a mere 13 times in 3 hours. But the mice who received high-potency maca had sex 67 times. "Maca has long been talked about as a sexual enhancer, but this is the first time it's been scientifically shown," says Qun Yi Zheng, Ph.D., the author of the study, which was published in the journal *Urology*.

Trials testing maca on humans are already under way.

A Male Birth Control Pill?

Mice may also lead the way to a male birth control pill. Researchers at the University of Leicester in England reduced fertility rates in male mice by 90 percent by deactivating receptor proteins on the vas deferens, the sperm-carrying tube that is cut in a vasectomy. Scientists believe that drugs could be developed to inhibit the proteins. "A male pill might be a temporary vasectomy," says Catrin Pritchard, Ph.D., one of the researchers.

Dr. Pritchard says that it could take a number of years before a male birth control pill is available.

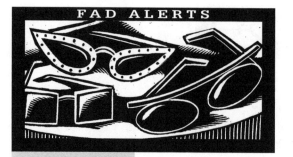

Proxeed Drink Mix

 An Italian company, Sigma-Tau Pharmaceuticals, is marketing Proxeed drink mix to fertility doctors and would-be fathers in the United States. It has allegedly been proven to "promote optimum sperm quality," which supposedly means that it improves the odds of a man fathering a child. The mix sells for $95 a month.

The chief ingredient in Proxeed is carnitine, a nutrient made by the liver and found in fish and milk. Sigma-Tau Pharmaceuticals cites eight European studies involving 342 men. Each man took 1 to 4 grams of carnitine daily for up to 6 months. In a few instances, sperm motility was reported to have doubled. In other cases, sperm counts were up by 80 percent. In one study of 20 men, five were able to get their wives pregnant.

But these small studies don't prove that carnitine had any positive effect, says Mark Sigman, M.D., a urologist at Brown University in Providence, Rhode Island, who is currently conducting a study on Proxeed. Most didn't use a placebo, and the one study that did (of 60 men) was too poorly designed to yield reliable results. "Sperm counts fluctuate, and they might have increased naturally even if these men had taken nothing," explains Dr. Sigman. "There's no biological reason carnitine would increase sperm production."

Peter Schlegel, M.D., a urologist at Cornell University in Ithaca, New York, agrees. "The only way to judge if a fertility treatment works is to see if it causes more pregnancies than a placebo," he says. "The few pregnancies that occurred during these small trials don't prove anything."

Veromax

Veromax contains L-arginine and other natural ingredients claimed to help trap blood in the penis for better erections. A 1-month supply of 60 pills (550 milligrams each) costs $80. The company has no scientific studies to back up the claim, and the urologist who sells it has had his medical license suspended.

Is it worth buying? No. "There is no research to support that impotent men have a deficiency in L-arginine in the first place, so ingesting more may not make a difference," says Laurence Levine, M.D., professor of urology at Rush-Presbyterian-St. Luke's Medical Center in Chicago.

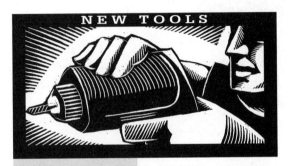

NEW TOOLS

A Better Treatment for Infertility

Varicocele Embolization

Nearly half of all men evaluated for infertility suffer from varicocele: swollen veins in the scrotum that can reduce sperm production. Now a new, nonsurgical procedure can quickly fix varicocele. During varicocele embolization, a thin tube is inserted into each vein, and steel plugs are used to block the blood flow that causes swelling. In a study at the University of British Columbia in Vancouver, fewer than 1 percent of men needed to repeat the procedure, compared with 12 percent to 16 percent of patients who had had surgery. Embolization patients also recovered 2 weeks sooner. Varicocele embolization is now available at most U.S. hospitals.

Faster Herpes Test

Pockit HSV 2 Rapid Test

Gone are the days when you had to sweat out the results of a herpes blood or swab test for up to 2 weeks. The Pockit HSV 2 Rapid Test detects herpes in a blood sample in just 10 minutes. The test is manufactured by Diagnology and is available only in doctors' offices. If herpes is caught early enough, a vigorous round of drug therapy can eliminate or lessen symptoms (such as lesion outbreaks) for as long as the patient is taking the medication.

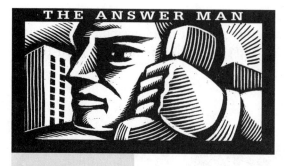

The Downside of Doin' It

I came down with a urinary tract infection after a long, sexy weekend with my girlfriend. We've been together for a year, and this has never happened before. How did she get the infection? Is she cheating on me?
—D. H., Knoxville, Tenn.

We strongly suspect she got her infection by having sex—with you. "During intercourse, bacteria can be forced up a woman's urethra," says Kathleen Fitzgerald, M.D., of Brown University School of Medicine in Providence, Rhode Island. "If the bacteria travel into the bladder, an infection can result." Making love more than once in a single day or night can irritate the urethra, increasing her chances of infection.

To avoid infecting herself and then you, your girlfriend should make a bathroom stop before and after sex. That way, even if some bacteria reach the bladder, they won't be there long enough to multiply. If she's using a diaphragm, she might want to switch to another form of birth control. Diaphragms can put pressure on the urethra, making an infection more likely. And using lots of lubrication during sex—her own or an over-the-counter product such as K-Y Liquid—will reduce friction and decrease the wear and tear down there. If she continues to suffer from infections, her doctor may prescribe an oral antibiotic such as Bactrim to take immediately after sex.

The Honeymoon's Over

I've been married for 6 years. My wife and I used to have sex every night, but now I'm lucky if it's once a week, or sometimes once a month. Am I normal?
—G. T., Wilmington, Del.

We hate to break it to you, but your grandfather got it more than you do. Sixty years ago, the average married guy in his thirties probably had sex about three times per week, says Domeena Renshaw, M.D., founder of the Loyola University sexual dysfunction clinic. Now, that same 30-year-old is lucky to average about seven times a month—or barely twice a week. The reason? Today there are dual-career marriages—and ESPN. To get your average back up, don't argue or complain about the lack of frequency. Instead, tell her, "I would really love if we had sex tonight." That gives her a chance to react, rather than be defensive.

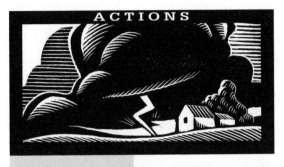

Some aspects of that incredible thing known as sex should remain a mystery. The hows and whys of attraction, for example. But it's no mystery that a good lover is a knowledgeable lover. With that in mind, here's a collection of techniques and tips to keep you at the top of your game.

1. Imitate the butterfly. No two ways about it—your groin muscles work overtime in the sack. The best way to keep them flexible and avoid embarrassing and untimely muscle cramps is with a butterfly stretch, says Eric Gronbech, Ph.D., professor of physical education at Chicago State University who researches the link between fitness and libido. Lie flat on your back in bed, knees bent, feet flat on the mattress. Pull your heels toward your buttocks; now turn your ankles so the soles and heels of your feet are touching one another. Your knees should naturally point out to the sides. Now let gravity do its thing—let your knees slowly drop toward the bed. When they're as far apart as possible, hold for a count of 10, then bring your knees back up. Relax, repeat twice.

2. Don't take Viagra as dessert. Wait at least 90 minutes after a lavish dinner to take your dose of Viagra. High-fat foods prevent you from fully absorbing it. "If I hear a man say Viagra didn't work for him, it's usually because he took it too soon after a fatty meal," says Ken Goldberg, M.D., a urologist in Dallas. You can also take Viagra 90 minutes before eating. It'll be absorbed by the time you eat, and you'll have 12 hours to enjoy the effects.

3. If you're looking to please her, think low. No, lower, smart guy. Scores of women say that, when it comes to an explosively pleasurable sensory experience, a good foot rub ranks right up there with nipple stimulation and oral sex. If you want to be a man who knows how to please women, you'd better learn to give good foot. Here's how, according to Gordon Inkeles, a masseur in Bayside, California, and author of *The New Sensual Massage*.

- Take her foot in your hand, begin kneading with your fingertips, and work your way from the ankle to the toes, all the while kneading both the inside and the outside of the foot.
- When you're through with that, push the tip of your thumb or all four knuckles into the depression of her arch, again with gentle pressure.
- Same again, this time using your thumb or knuckle to put pressure on her heel.
- One by one, take each toe and give it a slow, delicate tug.

4. **Take a seat.** For a variation on the traditional sitting position, first find a sturdy chair. You might prefer a cushioned seat as well. Now, instead of her straddling you, have her take the sitting equivalent of the spoons position. She's on your lap, with her back facing you. You enter her from the rear, and now have your hands free to hold her, massage her, or wander pretty much anywhere on her body the two of you want to go. If her legs are long enough (that is, the chair's legs are short enough), she can supply some of the thrust, but if not, the two of you will have to get yourselves into a coordinated rhythm of push and pull.

5. **Think in twos.** If you want to turn your short sprints into a marathon love session, double up on the condoms. Even if pregnancy is the farthest thing from your mind, and you've been in a monogamous relationship for years, there's something to be said for the desensitizing nature of condoms. Some extra layers of latex could make the difference in lasting longer. So if you want an easy way to stay stronger longer, put on two condoms. Some men find the latex layers and the firmness of the condom ring keep them erect.

6. **Wait for the signal.** If you think your success with a potential mate hinges on the cleverness of your opening line, think again. According to Monica Moore, Ph.D., a professor of psychology at Webster University in St. Louis who has been studying courtship since 1978, women have already sized you up and made a decision about you before you can saunter over and use that clever opening line you've been saving. In fact, for better success at a singles bar, Dr. Moore suggests concentrating on women who are sending positive signals to you. She's identified 52 "flirting gestures." Here are her top five:

- Eyebrow flash: An exaggerated raising of the eyebrows of both eyes for a couple seconds, followed by a rapid lowering to the normal position. Often combined with a smile and eye contact.

- Lip lick: This gesture's very common. Some women use only a single-lip lick, wetting the upper or lower lip, while others run the tongue around the entire lip area.
- Short, darting glance: Usually occurs in bouts, with an average of three glances per bout.
- Hair flip: She pushes her fingers through her hair. Some women make only one hand movement, others stroke their hair.
- Coy smile: A sort of half-smile, showing little if any tooth, combined with a downward gaze or eye contact that is very brief.

7. **For ultimate kissing, think ears and neck.** Sure, the mouth is arousing. But a lot of women get even jumpier when they have their earlobes kissed, tongued, sucked, or lightly nibbled. One good technique is to gently tug on the lobe with your lips, then slowly work your way up to the ear itself and insert your tongue, like a swab, with slow circular motions. Soft breathing into her ear can also be quite a turn-on.

Another pleasure point is her neck, usually in the front, near the base. Again, try gentle kissing, followed by sucking, licking, and soft biting. If she picks her neck up a little bit, she's telling you that you've hit a good spot, so stick around a while. If she lowers it, move on.

8. **Make her an offer she can't refuse.** If you nag and downright beg, and your woman still remains tight-lipped about her sexual fantasies, do this first—stop nagging and begging. It's demeaning. Instead, give her a challenge. Tell her you'll do anything she wants in the bedroom for 1 hour, suggests Helen Fisher, Ph.D., research associate in the department of anthropology at Rutgers University in New Brunswick, New Jersey, and author of *Anatomy of Love*. Her response may be for you to paint the walls, but it also might get those wheels turning in her head. "Try it and find out what happens," Dr. Fisher advises. "Most couples who are sexually bored probably know very little about each other's fantasies and how to play into them."

9. **Knead to succeed.** The man who knows how to give a good massage is always in demand. So brush up on the different strokes involved. The most common stroke is *effleurage*, which uses the fingers and palm in long, gliding strokes that go toward the heart. Use it on the longer muscles like those in her back and legs. Then there's *petrissage*, a squeezing/compressing/kneading motion that rolls muscles across the grain. It works well on shorter muscles, like the shoulders, sides of the back, and triceps. Use deeper, firmer strokes to reduce stress and improve circulation. Save your soft, light strokes for a more arousing feel.

10. **Get visual.** An overwhelming number of men (93 percent) and women (81 percent) love to watch their partners undress, according to the landmark *Sex in America* survey. So learn how to incorporate some visual stimuli into your sex life. One of the easiest ways is to strip for each other. Sounds simple enough, but not enough couples take advantage of the potential this simple act offers for erotic scenarios, says Robert Birch, Ph.D., a psychologist who specializes in marriage and sex therapy and author of *Male Sexual Endurance*. "Try to catch her from a different angle," he says. "Encourage her to let you catch a peek here and there, as if she didn't know you were looking." Flashing and the striptease scenario are there for the exploiting, so why settle for just kicking off your clothes as though you were in a locker room?

11. **Learn a new position to last longer.** Experiment with different positions during intercourse to find one that allows you maximum control. In her work with men, Barbara Keesling, Ph.D., a California sex therapist and author of *How to Make Love All Night*, has found that one position seems to work best for ejaculatory control: a kind of modified missionary position. The woman lies on her back, perhaps with a small pillow under her back for comfort. Her legs are raised in the air, knees bent, and the man is on his knees between her legs. "The key to this position is that the man uses his knees instead of his arms to support most of his weight," she explains. By minimizing muscle tension in this way, he's able to use his PC muscles better. "Most men tell me this is the position with which they have their greatest success," she says.

12. **Talk dirty when she least expects it.** At the opera, in an art gallery, at the public library—these are common places where talk is strictly forbidden. What better place for talking dirty to one another? "It's the forbidden aspect," says Dr. Keesling, "You're not supposed to talk at all in the library or during 'Pomp and Circumstance.' So for some people, hearing sexy talk in so-called forbidden environments is especially arousing."

13. **Backache? Think spoons.** Your sex life doesn't need to stop if you or your partner is suffering from back pain. Try the "spoons" position: You both lie on your sides, you behind your mate, and you enter her from behind. This way, you're both resting, there's very little muscle strain, and it's easy to control the position of your back. For added comfort, place pillows between the knees of either of you.

14. **Tantalize her with your touches.** Shun routine in your touches as you would in anything else in your relationship. That means, among other things, shifting the intensity of your touches as the occasion warrants. Touch intensities can even be correlated to car gears, according to Barry McCarthy, Ph.D., a Washington, D.C., psychologist for the Washington Psychological Center and author of *Male Sexual Awareness*. First gear: affectionate touching, fully clothed. Second gear: semi-sexual touching, semi-clothed. Third gear: playful sexual touching, clothing optional. Fourth gear: sexual touching to orgasm. Overdrive: sexual touching during genital intercourse. "Learn to value all five gears," advises Dr. McCarthy.

15. **Take a breath.** In the heat of the moment, you start breathing heavy, your heart starts racing, and everything moves faster, including the time it'll take to ejaculate. To avoid fast-forwarding through the good parts, concentrate on taking long, slow, deep breaths. This gives you better oxygen flow and helps equalize everything even when you're in the midst of some scorching sex.

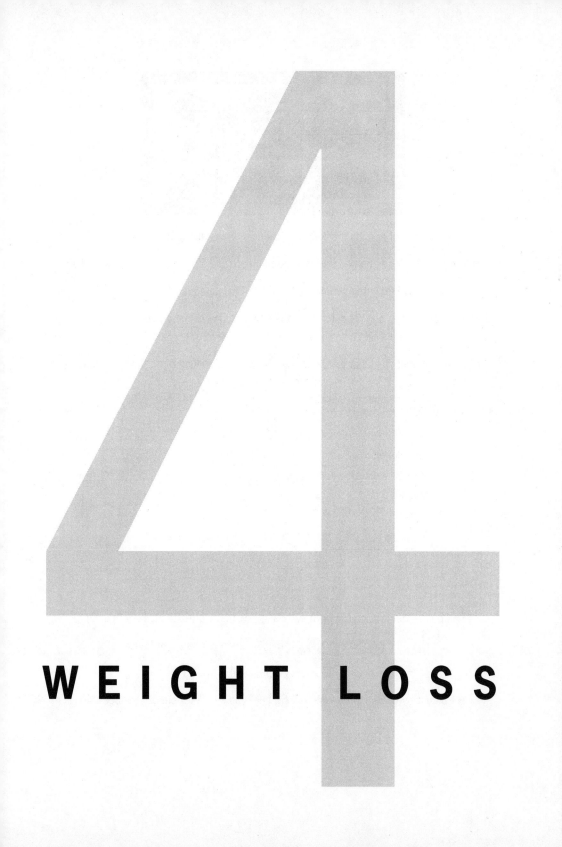

4

WEIGHT LOSS

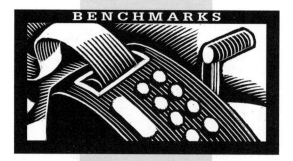

■ Number of pounds the average American gains during holiday time: 10

■ Number of calories burned by a 180-pound man for 1 hour of gutter cleaning: 409

■ Percentage chance that body fat is inherited: 25 to 40

■ Number of calories a 200-pound guy can eat in one day and still lose 1 pound a week if he walks a half-hour at a moderate pace daily: 2,580

■ Number of pounds lost in 1 year as a result of doing nothing more than 2 minutes of pushups everyday: 2.5

■ Number of calories burned by carrying a quart of water in your briefcase for 20 minutes: 96

■ Calories in a 16-ounce bottle of cranberry-grape blend: 340

■ Calories in a McDonald's Filet-o-Fish: 450

■ Calories in a McDonald's basic burger: 225

■ Minutes it takes to burn 31 calories dancing: 5

■ Calories in black coffee: 10

■ Calories in a café latte: 210

■ Pounds lost in one year from switching from café lattes to black coffee: 21

■ Calories saved by eating a filet mignon instead of a porterhouse: 122

■ Grams of fat saved: 16

■ Percent by which blotting and rinsing beef can knock fat out of your beef: 50

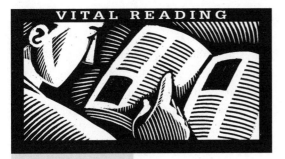

VITAL READING

The World's Best Weight-Loss Machine

For the ultimate weight-loss workout, rediscover your bike.

If you really want to shed your gut, pick up the first piece of fitness equipment you ever owned: your bike. Not only will cycling free you from the senses-dulling stair-climber routine, but it won't pound your joints or jiggle your gut the way running will. And done right, it can burn more calories than either.

To get fit fast, you need to ride so that you burn the maximum amount of calories and fat while steering clear of injuries. Here are nine strategies from the country's top cycling authorities.

Ride at least 4 days a week. Consistency rules when it comes to losing weight on the bike, says Edmund Burke, Ph.D., author of *Serious Cycling*. To lose a pound or two a week, aim for a minimum of three short rides of 30 to 60 minutes each during the week, and one longer trip of 1 to 2 hours on the weekend. If you haven't been on your bike for a while, stick to shorter rides until you're in good enough condition for a long one, Dr. Burke advises.

Here's what your minimum weekly workout should look like if you're riding a road bike. (You might want to get a Camelbak hydration bladder, the look-Ma-no-hands way to refuel with water on the road.)

- Monday: 45 minutes at moderate intensity (5 to 7 on an exertion scale of 10)
- Wednesday: 30 minutes of hills or flats at high intensity (exertion rate of 8)
- Friday: 45 minutes at moderate intensity (exertion rate of 5 to 7)
- Saturday: 1 to 2 hours at moderate intensity (exertion rate of 5 to 7)

To build muscle while you're riding, add these drills to your workout twice a week, recommends Chris Carmichael, former head coach of the U.S. Olympic Cycling Team and currently Lance Armstrong's coach.

- Power starts. Start at a very low speed (almost stopped) on a flat road. Put your bike in its biggest gear and begin hammering as hard as you can, out of the saddle, for 10 to 12 seconds or 8 to 10 pedal strokes. Recover for a few minutes and repeat.

• Stomp intervals. On flat terrain, start rolling in your largest gear until you reach 15 to 20 mph. Then, remaining in your saddle, pedal as hard as you can for about 20 seconds. Make sure you pull through the bottom of the pedal stroke and smoothly stomp down during the downstroke. Allow at least 5 minutes of recovery time between efforts.

Stay in the range. Most guys jump on their bikes and start hammering like they're Lance Armstrong, says Carmichael. That kind of all-out riding pushes your heart rate into the anaerobic range, so your body can't send oxygen to your muscles fast enough to burn fat. A recent article in the *Journal of Strength and Conditioning Research* concluded that fat oxidation—the rate at which you burn stored fat for fuel—peaks at about 60 percent of your maximum heart rate. "I coach riders to train just above that, at 65 to 75 percent, for the best overall fitness benefits," says Carmichael.

The most accurate way to tell whether you're riding in the right range is to calculate your maximum heart rate (220 minus your age) and strap on a heart-rate monitor when you ride. But you can also judge just by the way you feel. Rate your exertion on a scale of 1 to 10, with 1 being a light spin and 10 on the verge of blowing up. Try to stay between 5 and 7.

When time is short, step up your workout. Opening up the throttle once a week can be smart, too, especially if your time is limited, says Dr. Burke. "You burn more calories per minute riding at a higher intensity; you just can't ride as long," he says. If you can ride for only 30 minutes on a particular day, take your heart rate up to between 75 percent and 85 percent of your maximum (about an 8 on the exertion scale).

Stop coasting. Cycling at 15 mph burns about 650 calories an hour. "But that's only if you're pedaling," notes Dr. Burke. "Coasting doesn't burn many more calories than sitting in a recliner clicking the remote." To keep pedaling consistently, shift into a higher gear on easier terrain. "You'll burn twice as many calories as you would half-pedaling and half-coasting, and you'll lose weight faster."

Use your low gears on flats and uphills. Riding in a high gear feels more manly, but you'll save your knees and burn more calories by using a lower gear (a smaller chainring) and spinning quickly, the way the pros do, says Barney King, a U.S. Cycling Federation certified elite coach. "Spinning keeps you in that premium aerobic range. You burn fat without becoming fatigued." Aim for a cadence of 80 to 100 revolutions per minute. To determine your cadence, count the number of times your right leg hits the bottom of the pedal stroke in a 10-second period. Then multiply that number by six.

Sit down when going up. The quickest way to increase the intensity of your workout is to take it vertical, says Dr. Burke. "Hills burn a lot of calories in a short time." Adding hard hills to your itinerary will also make you stronger and faster—and therefore able to burn more calories—on the flats. "To climb most efficiently, drop into an easy low gear and keep spinning at no less than 60 to 70 rpm while seated," says Dr. Burke. "Standing drains energy."

Leave the beaten path. You don't see many fat mountain-bike riders. An hour of off-road riding burns about 600 calories and works your whole body, not just your legs. "There's more resistance on the trails, so you expend more energy," says Carmichael. You're building your upper-body muscles as you pull up over rocks and logs.

Restock your cells with a sports drink. After a hard ride, the glycogen, or stored fuel, in your muscles is low. You have about 20 minutes to replenish it or risk ravenously overeating later and jeopardizing your weight-loss goals, says Dr. Burke. Your best plan, he says, is to grab a sports drink that contains carbohydrates and protein in a 4-to-1 ratio. The protein helps repair your muscles, and the carbohydrates refuel them. "This is the step men forget," says Carmichael. "That's why they end up stuffing down $20 worth of Taco Bell in the evening and wondering why they aren't losing weight."

Eat the right food at the right time. Professional cyclists eat breakfasts that would put a lumberjack to shame. Yet they stay as skinny as their tires. "Sure, the number of hours they train helps, but the real secret is how they time their eating," says Nancy Clark, R.D., author of *Nancy Clark's Sports Nutrition Guidebook.*

Most men eat a light breakfast and lunch, go out and ride hard, then eat a pound of pasta before bedtime. "That's counterproductive," says Clark. "You should eat a big meal early in the day. A large bowl of cereal, an orange, and a bagel for breakfast, along with a comfortable lunch, will let you enjoy your ride without running on empty. Then you can replenish yourself after the ride with a high-carbohydrate snack, and eat appropriately throughout the rest of the day. With the exercise and the subsequent increase in your metabolism," notes Clark, "you'll still burn more calories than you've taken in, and you'll lose weight."

Wacky Weight-Loss Schemes (And the Hidden Wisdom behind Them)

There's more than one way to lose weight, as these four men discovered. Learn how—and why—their plans worked.

It's a sad fact that visionaries are usually mocked in their own time. When Alexander Graham Bell told his bar buddies about a device that could carry the human voice thousands of miles, they probably laughed and tossed beer nuts at him. When Albert Einstein first babbled on about relativity, his friends no doubt shook their heads and mumbled something about "Al finding a real job." When Bill Gates first spoke of Windows . . . well, actually Windows sounded like a pretty good idea.

Submitted for your approval: four modern-day visionaries who have discovered their own secrets for losing weight. You, too, might be tempted to mock and throw beer nuts at these men. A diet based on eating hoagies every day? Come on. A diet revolving around a mysterious ethnic soup?

You may be surprised to learn what was discovered when these fellows and their menus were submitted to two nutrition experts: Anne Fletcher, R.D., who has tracked more than 200 weight-loss success stories for her *Thin for Life* book series, and Tina Ruggiero, R.D., a New York City dietitian. They were able to offer expert advice on how to make even these singularly freakish plans work for you.

The Strange Facts Concerning Subway

Meet Jared, a 20-year-old college student at Indiana University who had a John Candy-esque weight problem—and by John Candy-esque, we mean that his parents feared he wouldn't live to see his 35th birthday. Jared was a whopping 425 pounds, with a size-60 waist. He ate anything and everything, especially fast food and pizza.

When Jared moved to a new dorm room, he found that it was right next door to a Subway sandwich shop. He looked at the sign advertising the "Seven Under Six Grams of Fat" menu, and thought, "This is what I need." Each day, Jared ate only two sandwiches from the low-fat menu: a foot-long veggie and a 6-inch turkey, with no cheese and no mayo, but tons of lettuce, green peppers, banana peppers, jalapeño peppers, and pickles, and a bit of spicy mustard. Aside from diet soft drinks, nothing else passed Jared's lips.

Over the course of a year, Jared lost a flabbergasting 245 pounds. He's currently 180 and has been maintaining a size-34 waist.

Why it worked: "Portion control," says Fletcher. "You can do the same thing by having Slim-Fast twice a day. But Jared found something that was easy and convenient—somebody made it for him—and he liked it, so it worked." And, of course, Jared didn't have to worry about counting calories, since they never—ever—varied. Furthermore, Ruggiero points out that the lettuce and peppers gave Jared a good dose of fiber. "High fiber keeps you full and acts like a brush, binding to fat and sweeping it out of your intestines," she explains. Thanks for the image, Tina.

How to make it work for you: If you don't want to count calories but you lack Jared's ability to eat the same damned thing day after day after day, try what Ruggiero calls the "balanced plate." Make sure it's mostly carbohydrates (one big baked potato, a dinner roll) and vegetables. Then include about 4 to 6 ounces (about the size of a deck of cards) of protein, such as fish, chicken, turkey, and a tiny bit of fat (margarine on the potato).

Keep in mind that you don't have to take the Subway to practice portion control when you want fast food. There are plenty of other places that offer items that are low in fat. Dig Wendy's? You're in luck. Taco Bell? Ditto. Big Daddy Don's House of Fried Animals? Sorry.

The Shocking Enigma of Cuban Weight-Loss Soup

Paul, a 5-foot-7, 197-pound computer programmer, tried several different weight-loss plans but usually ended up gaining everything back in a weekend. "I pretty much ate what I wanted, although I had a healthy diet," says Paul. His one vice is beer, which he, shockingly enough, enjoys a lot.

Then Paul's best friend's wife introduced him to a strange, exotic potion: traditional "Cuban Weight-Loss Soup," made from celery, cabbage, and onions. According to Paul, this soup works because you burn more calories digesting the celery in the soup than the celery contains. "You can eat it hot or cold—but it will take the weight off fast." Paul ate salads and fruit along with at least two bowls of soup per day.

In just 1 week, Paul lost 7 pounds! He's currently trying to crack the 190-pound barrier by exercising when he's not eating soup.

Why it worked: One thing's for sure: It had nothing to do with Paul's theory about celery taking more energy to digest than it supplies. "There's simply no evidence that it's true," says Fletcher. Besides, man cannot live on celery alone. That's why God created buffalo wings.

The real reason Paul lost 7 pounds in a week was because he ate soup, a lot of soup. A recent study at Pennsylvania State University found that subjects ate less when they were served chicken-and-rice soup than when they were served the same ingredients in casserole form. Since Paul was eating less, he was taking in fewer calories. Unfortunately, he was also taking in almost no protein. "A red flag goes up when I hear about people eating nothing but soup all day," says Ruggiero.

How to make it work for you: Along with protein and several other essential nutrients, there's something missing from Paul's soup diet: variety. As good as the Cuban Weight-Loss Soup may taste (we have our doubts), it wouldn't be too palatable or healthy after 3 weeks of slurping. Better to pick several soups that you like and work them into a balanced diet on a rotating basis. Unless your favorite soups are Cream of Mushroom, Cream of Clam Chowder, and Cream of Heavy Thick Cream, you should notice the pounds slipping away.

The Creepy Caffeine Conundrum

Following in the tradition of countless accidental inventors before him, Mitch, a 49-year-old government employee, stumbled onto his discovery. He wasn't trying to lose weight—he was just trying to get rid of the blasted headaches that had been troubling him. On the advice of a friend of his, a doctor, Mitch decided to cut caffeine out of his diet.

When Mitch quit caffeine, he thought he might calm down, but he didn't expect to slim down. But within 2 weeks, he noticed that he was dropping weight, and it continued for 4 to 6 weeks until he had lost a total of 14 pounds off his 5-foot-7 frame. "After that, I decided to capitalize on the results by trying to lose more weight," says Mitch. He gave up all dairy and most bread, stopped snacking, and switched from meat to fish.

One month after losing his first 14 pounds, Mitch clocked in at 150 pounds—way down from his original weight of 187. But three questions remained: Why? Why? Why?

Why it worked: Dumb luck. By cutting out all that coffee and soda, Mitch cut out as much as 4 pints of water weight a day. "Just 1 pint of water weighs 1 pound," explains Ruggiero. "That would explain why the weight loss didn't continue until he changed the rest of his diet—his body began to conserve fluid more efficiently in an attempt to stay hydrated."

As for the rest of Mitch's weight loss, it was a matter of simple calorie reduction. When Mitch stopped drinking 4 cups of coffee a day, he gave up not only his headaches but 300 calories in creamer as well.

How to make it work for you: Kick your coffee and soda habit, even if you're downing decaf and diet. Like Mitch, you'll experience pretty quick and dramatic weight loss. It won't last, but that's okay; the real payoff will come when you see what you looked like prior to packing on the pounds. "Losing a few pounds can be a powerful psychological motivator to lose even more weight," says Ruggiero.

The Freakish 4 O'Clock Fat-Melting Effect

Consider the case of Dan, an entomologist whose 220 pounds gravitated toward a 38-inch waist. "In this part of Texas, foods tend to be incredibly fattening," he says. To make things worse, Dan would find himself eating five meals a day—breakfast, lunch, an afterwork snack, dinner, and a late-night snack. He might have considered moving out of Texas, but instead he took some advice from his ex-girlfriend and started spending nights alone—that is, without food.

"My secret is no food after 4:00 P.M.," says Dan. "I can eat anything and everything for breakfast and lunch, or in the afternoon, but come 4 o'clock, my lips are sealed." Sometimes Dan would become hungry at night, but he would tell himself to hold on, and he'd reward himself in the morning. "There's a Burger King on the way to work," he says, laughing.

Five months and a backseat full of fast-food containers later, Dan weighed a svelte 180 pounds, and his waist had shrunk from 38 to 31 inches. Time to buy new pants!

Why it worked: Basically, Dan discovered a new way to stop being a pig. "He cut out two of his meals, and probably reduced his caloric intake by a third," says Ruggiero. "That would make anybody lose weight."

Time, however, was not of the essence: There was nothing magical about cutting out those calories after 4:00 P.M. It wouldn't have mattered if his cutoff was 5:00, 6:00, or 7:00. There's little support for the theory that eating your calories during the day is any better than eating them at night, says Fletcher. Besides, you're just setting yourself up for the kind of disaster that befell the Hindenberg. All it would take is one call from a buddy to go out for a couple of beers and burgers and blammo! Goodbye, diet. Oh, the humanity!

How to make it work for you: Uh, don't. Fast food every morning on the way to work? Sure, if you don't mind a trip to the emergency room on the way home from work that night. "Granted, you might find yourself at your ideal weight," says Ruggiero, "but you'll be making yourself a prime candidate for a heart attack." Taking pounds off your body should never mean taking years off your life.

About the only lesson to take away from Dan's story is to try to stick to three meals a day. That means making sure that your afternoon and late-evening snacks are just that—snacks. And small ones at that. In case you're wondering, an afternoon pick-me-up of 2 dozen Cool Ranch Doritos washed down with a 20-ounce Coke is a 530-calorie meal. And don't try to squeeze in all of your meals before some arbitrary deadline. Stop at 4:00 P.M., and sooner or later you'll give in to your demonic hunger pangs and end up bingeing at 10:00.

The moral of these tales from the underbelly of the weight-loss world? Perhaps it's that even if a strange diet works for you, it may not be for the reasons you think. (Even worse, your diet may be shortchanging you nutritionally at the same time it stains the upholstery in the new VW.) Or maybe it's that personal motivation can be an incredibly powerful tool—when coupled with sound nutritional advice.

Break Out of Hibernation

If your exercise and good eating plans have disappeared with the sun, follow these suggestions to get back on track.

As winter wears on, the days get shorter, the bowl games get longer, and the pizzas get bigger.

Call it human hibernation. It's one of the things that link us to our cute mammal friends—chipmunks and raccoons and Governor Jesse Ventura. "Animals respond to light and temperature cues," says Greg Florant, Ph.D., of Colorado State University in Fort Collins, who studies hibernating animals. These cues compel bears, for example, to store 50 percent of their body weight as fat in preparation for the long, cold nights of winter. Does that remind you of anyone?

It should. Most of us spend our winters like giant, hairy carnivores, sleeping more, eating more—and exercising less.

But when the time comes to leave the cave, you need an exit strategy. Try these 19 exercise and fitness strategies to help get you out of your bear suit.

The Damage: Not As Bad As You Think

Don't worry about the long-term effects of a winter layoff. There really aren't any. "Your fitness will ebb and flow, like everything else in your body. In the long run, it's really irrelevant if you miss a couple of weeks here and there," says Bryant Stamford, Ph.D., an exercise physiologist at the University of Louisville.

Just Show Up

Longer nights actually have a physiological effect on men's bodies. A lack of the hormone melatonin (its production is linked to duration of daylight) makes us sluggish, and we spend our days covered up in layers of bulky clothing, making it easy to hide our spreading love handles.

But there's one place where people aren't covered up, where the lights are bright, and where we feel a surge of adrenaline just by walking in the door—and it's not a maternity ward. "Just go to a gym," suggests Michael George, a trainer in Los Angeles. "Your mentality will shift back. You'll see people who look good, and that'll motivate you." Buy a pass and spend the whole darn day there. Don't push yourself. Try out every aerobic and strength machine—and play with all the buttons and settings—until you know how everything works. The next time you go, you won't be stuck doing the same old routine, like you did last year.

The First Step: Gooooal!

What's the first thing most of us do to get back into shape? According to Liz Neporent, C.S.C.S., a trainer and coauthor of *Fitness for Dummies*, we get stupid. We join a gym, or buy a $3,000 treadmill, or hire a $100-an-hour personal trainer, all without any idea of what we ultimately want to accomplish. But we need goals, not gadgets. "Don't start with, 'I want to get in shape and lose weight,'" says Neporent. That first goal has to be specific: lose 2 inches off your waist, drop 10 pounds, get ready for a summer basketball league, bench-press 200 pounds.

Once you have a specific goal, the next step is to give yourself time to accomplish it. Tell yourself you're going to lose 2 inches or 10 pounds in 6 to 8 weeks. "It's hard to see progress from day to day, so this way you always know if you're reaching your goals or falling short," says Alwyn Cosgrove, C.S.C.S., a trainer in North Hills, California.

Now, Make a Plan

Just as you wouldn't rent a Porsche to haul your furniture, you shouldn't go into the gym and start pumping iron if your goal is to lose your gut. All exercise is good for something, but no exercise is good for everything.

If you want to lose inches: Combine weight training, cardiovascular exercise, and a smarter diet. A 1999 study found that guys who did all three lost 22 pounds in 12 weeks, and virtually all the weight lost was fat. We'll get into more specifics on this program later.

If you want to lose pounds: Focus on food and aerobic exercise. "You're looking at about 80 percent diet and 20 percent exercise," says Dr. Stamford. Exercise is important—the nation's most successful weight-droppers work off about 2,800 calories a week, according to the National Weight Control Registry—but the best exercise is the two-armed table push-back. When it comes to losing weight, diet gets you there faster.

Here's why: Walking or running a mile burns roughly 100 calories. To lose a pound of fat, you need to burn 3,500 calories. That's 35 miles per pound, or almost a marathon and a 10-miler combined. That'll make the turkey sandwich on dry toast go down easier, right?

If you only want to build strength: Hit the weight room. Don't severely limit your calories, and go easy on the aerobic exercise, too. Both of those could lower your testosterone, making it tougher to add strength.

If you want to prepare for a sport: Work on skills (shooting, hitting, throwing), and the type of endurance the sport requires. For example, basketball and tennis require short bursts of speed; running longer distances slowly won't get you ready for that.

Also focus on flexibility. Mark Noble, C.S.C.S., flexibility consultant for the Duke University basketball team, found that the team's performance improved about 30 percent over a 2-year period when he had the players begin a program of simple stretches. His favorite full-body stretch:

Squat down and try to get your tailbone as close to your heels as possible while keeping your feet flat on the floor. Place your elbows inside your knees and push your knees apart. Now lean forward a little farther. This one stretch hits your Achilles tendons, lower back, and groin muscles.

Choose Your Weapons

It's one thing to say, "I need to do aerobic exercise," or "I really should lift weights." It's another thing not to hate every second of it. Three approaches to try:

Distraction: "Distract yourself with some sort of entertainment," Neporent suggests. Tell yourself you can only read your favorite mystery author when you're on the recumbent bike. Make the treadmill your Louis Rukheyser hour. At high-end gyms, you can surf the Web while on a stationary bike.

Aspiration: In the most soul-numbing moments of the most boring meetings of your career, what do you wish you could be doing instead? Climbing a mountain? Hitting a home run? Starring in your own straight-to-video martial-arts movie? Work with that. Schedule a vacation that involves hiking and climbing. Or sign up for an entry-level karate class. Then do whatever cardio-vascular exercise and strength training you need to get in shape for it. Give yourself a reasonable time frame—close enough to see, far enough away to make it possible. One month should do it.

Recreation: No rule says that exercise has to be plodding around a track or smelting iron in a room full of muscleheads. Recreational sports burn calories, too. Say you play three rounds of golf a week, walking and pulling your clubs with a handcart, which would be about 15 miles of walking, or 1,500 calories burned. That's the American College of Sports Medicine's recommended minimum to improve your health.

Some other ways a 185-pound man can burn 1,500 calories in a week without feeling miserable:

Doubles tennis: 3 hours

Fly-fishing: 3 hours

Softball: 3½ hours

Using power tools: 3 hours

Lawn mowing (no, not a riding mower): 4 hours

Drumming: 4½ hours

Vigorous sex: 12 hours

Driving a drag racer: 3 hours

Start at the Halfway Point

Your first week back, attempt to do only half of what you did before. Work out with half the weight. Walk or run half the miles. Hit half as many golf balls or baseballs, or shoot half as many jumpers.

After a couple of weeks, you may feel the temptation to start pushing yourself. Don't. Your feet, knees, elbows, and shoulders aren't ready for the pounding, even if your muscles feel great and your stamina seems to be returning. "Your joints and connective tissues won't give you any feedback until there's a problem," says Dr. Stamford.

Instead, increase your miles and speed and weights lifted by 10 percent a week, tops. If you start your program with half of what you were doing before, you can get back to two-thirds within a month. In 2 months, you'll be better than ever.

Eat Better

Most of us fall off all our wagons at least once. When we stop exercising, we stop eating carefully and start drinking sloppily. Here's something you can do tomorrow to eat lighter and healthier: Pack your own lunch.

"The more you eat out, the less control you have over your food, and the more likely you are to overeat," says Mary Flynn, R.D., Ph.D., a nutrition researcher at Brown University in Providence, Rhode Island. Even when you order just a sandwich at a deli, you eat more food than you'd ever make for yourself.

If you want to lose weight fast:

- Go off the juice. "Sometimes a guy can just stop drinking sodas and juices and drop 5 pounds in a month," says Flynn.
- Stay away from bars. Energy bars, anyway. Or protein drinks, energy gels, or any of the other high-calorie additives that come with workouts these

days. Unless you're trying to gain weight, the fat around your waist is all the energy you need for moderate workouts.

• Make friends with fruits. Add a fruit to each meal, and a vegetable to lunch and dinner. You'll feel fuller and eat less at your next snack or meal.

And, if you're really, really serious about losing weight, eat like Mother Teresa did. "If men eliminated meat and beer, they could drop 10 pounds in a month," Flynn says. A less radical measure is to use meat as a condiment, rather than the main attraction: Make it part of a sandwich or a salad, or use it in a pasta sauce.

The Gut-Shrinking Workout

Okay, you've decided on a specific goal and have taken some simple steps toward revamping your diet. It's now time to get on to the specifics of your workout program. First, take out a tape measure. Now measure your waist around your belly button. Next, suck in your waist until it's 2 inches smaller. That's what the average guy gets on this program, according to Michael Wood, C.S.C.S., owner of the Sports Performance Group in Cambridge, Massachusetts.

Weights: Do each workout twice a week. The weights specified here are just suggestions; they may be too light or heavy. Just make sure you improve each week.

Cardiovascular: Before each weight workout, do 30 minutes of cardiovascular exercise at a challenging intensity. Three other days a week, do 60 minutes of cardiovascular exercise at a slightly lower intensity; you can do this all at once or break it up—30 minutes before work and 30 minutes after, 20 minutes three times a day, and so forth.

DUMBBELL SQUAT

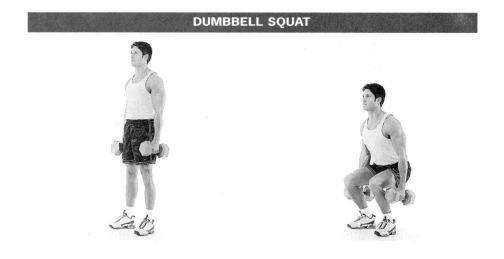

DUMBBELL STEPUP

DUMBBELL LUNGE

ONE-ARM BENT-OVER ROW

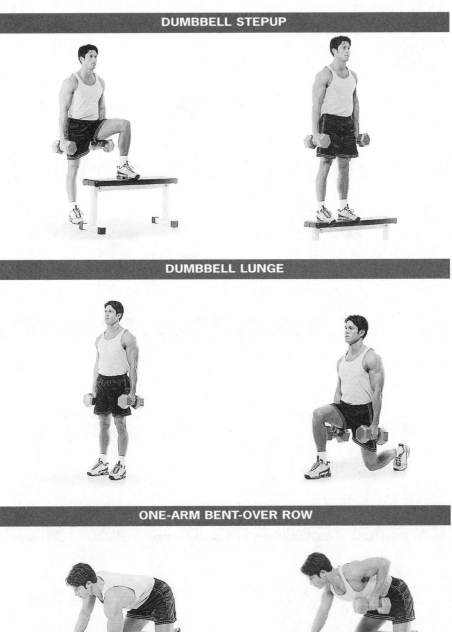

PUSHUP

DECLINE PUSHUP

DUMBBELL BENCH PRESS

DUMBBELL PUSH-PRESS

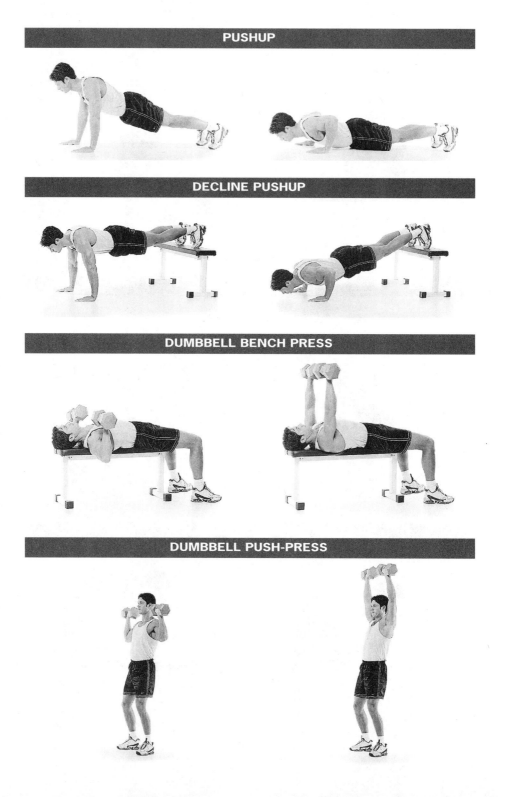

Exercise	Weight	Sets	Repetitions
Week 1			
Dumbbell squat	15	1	15
One-arm bent-over row	20	1	15
Pushup	Body	1	15
Dumbbell push-press	15	1	12
Week 2			
Dumbbell squat	20	2	12
One-arm bent-over row	25	2	12
Pushup	Body	2	12
Dumbbell push-press	20	2	12
Week 3			
Dumbbell squat	20	3	12
One-arm bent-over row	25	3	12
Pushup	Body	3	12
Dumbbell push-press	20	3	12
Week 4			
Dumbbell stepup	15	3	12
One-arm bent-over row	25	3	12
Pushup	Body	3	12
Dumbbell push-press	20	3	12
Week 5			
Dumbbell stepup	20	3	10
One-arm bent-over row	30	3	10
Decline pushup	Body	3	10
Dumbbell push-press	20	3	10
Week 6			
Dumbbell stepup	25	3	8
One-arm bent-over row	35	3	8*
Decline pushup	Body	3	10†
Dumbbell push-press	25	3	8

(continued)

Exercise	Weight	Sets	Repetitions
Week 7			
Dumbbell lunge	15	3	8
One-arm bent-over row	40	3	8*
Dumbbell bench press	30	3	10
Dumbbell push-press	25	3	10
Week 8			
Dumbbell lunge	20	3	8
One-arm bent-over row	45	3	6–8
Dumbbell bench press	30	3	10
Dumbbell push-press	25	3	10

*Hold the dumbbell in the "up" position for 3 seconds on each repetition.
†Hold your body in the "down" position for 3 seconds on each repetition.

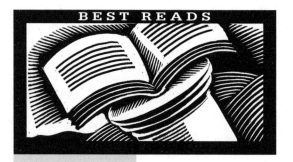

BEST READS

Fat City

Turkey frankfurters. Low-fat frozen meals. 2 percent milk. With all the low-fat products on the market these days, it should be a breeze to lose weight, right? As Dr. Ron and Nancy Goor explain in this excerpt adapted from Choose to Lose Weight-Loss Plan for Men: A Take-Control Program for Men with the Guts to Lose *(Houghton Mifflin), fat can be lurking in what appear to be innocent food choices. Read on to find out where fat may be creeping into your diet, and discover some healthier—and just as tasty—substitutes.*

Fat is everywhere. It is difficult to avoid. Turn on your television set and watch the melted cheese gently enfold a thick, juicy hamburger, or sweet, creamy chocolate swirl smoothly around a gooey nougat center, or cheese joyfully bubble atop a pizza crust. Drive through your town and count the fast-food restaurants as you whiz by. Take a good look at the dishes displayed behind the glass show-case in your office cafeteria. Fat! Fat! Fat!

And because fat is so available and convenient, Americans are getting fatter and fatter. Statistics show that more than 54 percent of Americans—97 million people—are overweight. Of those, 39 million are obese.

It's easy to do. Americans are eating out (much of it fast-food), carrying in, or popping high-fat convenience foods into the microwave. They are eating high-fat snacks and avoiding fruits and vegetables. Americans are driving more and walking less.

But this doesn't have to be you. You have the power to take control of the high-fat world around you. Once you know that fat is the culprit and where you can find it, you can root it out. You have the power. You can make educated choices. You can make lifestyle choices to reduce your exposure. You won't suffer. You can even splurge once in a while, since you'll know the cost.

In this chapter, we will briefly discuss fat-filled land mines and their lower-fat alternatives. But this generalized information is not enough. It is essential to look up fat calories in the Food Tables or on nutrition labels for every food you eat because fat content is not always obvious. Some is visible, like the strip of fat on a sirloin steak. But much is hidden, like the fat marbled throughout the steak and the fat added to processed frozen dinners.

Red Meats

Most of us were raised with the notion that you need to eat lots of protein to be healthy and fit. And what is usually considered the best source of protein? Red meat—beef, lamb, veal, and pork. Not true. Just as good sources are chicken, turkey, fish, seafood, and beans—and they are low in fat. Almost everyone gets enough protein no matter what their diet, and overeating protein can be dangerous to your health. And more than being a good source of protein, red meat is a super source of fat. Instead of building bulging biceps and triceps, eating lots of red meat builds bulging bellies, hips, and thighs. A lot of the fat is the worst kind—saturated fat. It's the kind that clogs your arteries and leads to heart attacks.

Even athletes no longer bulk up on steaks and eggs. Now they eat carbohydrates for energy.

For those of you who cannot envision life without a daily red meat fix, you can fit it into your diet. Obviously you can't afford a 10-ounce porterhouse steak

(540 fat calories) or two 3½-ounce lamb chops (530 fat calories) or 8 ounces of spareribs (616 fat calories) as daily fare, but if you plan for it and save up fat calories, an occasional red meat splurge can be budgeted in.

You may not believe it now, but if you limit your consumption of high-fat meats, you may even lose your taste for them after a while. A lineman from Virginia who had been following the *Choose to Lose Weight-Loss Plan for Men* for about 6 months, totally avoiding fast food, told us that he decided to give himself a birthday treat—a McDonald's quarter-pounder. He bought the sandwich and found it so greasy he couldn't eat it. Scientific studies have shown that it takes about 12 weeks to change from a high-fat to a low-fat taste.

Better Choices: Fish

If you want a steak, occasionally fit in a swordfish, tuna, or salmon steak. Although higher in fat than many fish, most of these big chunks of fish are lower in fat than cuts of beef, and in addition to being delicious, contain omega-3 polyunsaturated fats, which reduce the risks of heart disease and stroke by lowering high blood triglycerides and reducing blood clotting. At 10 fat calories per ounce for swordfish, 12 for tuna, and 9 to 27 for salmon depending on the type, these fish steaks are not as low-fat as many fish (cod is 2 fat calories per ounce, snapper 3 fat calories per ounce, and sole 3 fat calories per ounce), but the fat is a healthy fat. However, don't go overboard—even healthy fats are fattening.

Better Choices: Poultry

Chicken is a great substitute for beef and pork. It is also more versatile than beef. You can prepare chicken in a million tasty ways. At only 13 fat calories for a boneless, skinless chicken breast, chicken is a buy—fat-calorie-wise.

Even lower in fat at 2 fat calories per ounce, white-meat turkey can be turned into a multitude of scrumptious dishes. It is even delicious eaten plain.

Poultry

Although chicken has the potential to be a healthy choice, don't automatically equate chicken with low-fat. White-meat chicken prepared without skin and little added fat is a low-fat food, but chicken with the skin has a fat content approaching or even surpassing that of many cuts of beef. When fried, breaded, and deep-fried, or smothered in high-fat sauces, chicken joins the high-fat food brigade. Look at the chart below to see how easy it is to fatten up a chicken.

Preparation of Chicken Breast	Fat Calories
Roasted without skin	13
Roasted with skin, then skin removed	28
Roasted and eaten with skin	69
Fried with skin, flour coated	78
Fried with skin, batter dipped	166
KFC Extra Crispy	216
Chicken pot pie (Marie Callender's)	880

Turkey: Throw Away the Wrapping

Eat the turkey (white-meat turkey without the skin has 2 fat calories per ounce; dark meat without the skin has 9) but unless you have been banking fat calories for a Thanksgiving Day blowout, toss the skin. At 100 fat calories per ounce, even a little skin contains more fat than you need.

Chicken and Turkey Burgers

When you see chicken burger or turkey burger on a menu, don't automatically jump to order one. They may be lower in fat than a hamburger, but once the chef grinds in skin and fat, molds it into a burger, and fries it in oil, your poultry burger becomes a fat patty.

You also need to take care if you buy ground turkey at the grocery store. Ground turkey can be a good substitute for ground beef, but not if it is loaded with turkey skin and fat. Ground turkey can contain as much as 33 fat calories an ounce. Read the nutrition label if there is one; don't buy if there isn't.

Your best bet is to buy boneless chicken breasts without skin and grind your own meat in your food processor. Mix in some chopped carrots, celery, green pepper, onion, and some herbs, form patties, broil them, and you have a truly low-fat treat.

Redi-Serve Fat

The food industry is always up-to-the-minute in creating foods that will save us time, but at what expense? A new category of ready-made, prepared meats has cropped up in the market. But be sure to pick and choose carefully. For example, you can buy Redi-Serve breaded and cooked chicken patties (white meat) at a mind-boggling cost of 150 fat calories per patty. These patties have even more fat than the veal patties made by Redi-Serve.

Tyson makes roasted chicken that you just heat up. At first glance it looks pretty low in fat—25 fat calories for a chicken breast. That's only 12 more fat calories than if you roasted it yourself. Look again. With the skin, the chicken contains 120 fat calories a breast. Make sure you read every label carefully.

Duck: Super Splurge

A duck needs all that fat to keep it warm and afloat while it frolics in freezing water, but you don't. Half a duck with skin contains 975 fat calories—and that's without a sauce. However, if duck à l'orange is one of your absolute favorites in all the world, save up fat calories for a very, very, very special occasion and enjoy the treat.

Seafood

Snapper, shrimp, lobster, and sole—most plain, unadulterated fish or seafood contains 2 to 4 fat calories an ounce and can be a great low-fat choice. Once they start swimming around in the deep-fryer or butter or cream sauces, they need to be considered weight-gain and artery-clogging food.

Choose fish that has been baked, broiled, poached, or grilled with little or no fat for a delectable, guilt-free entrée.

A tip: Oil-packed tuna has 10 times as much fat as water-packed. A whole can of undrained tuna packed in water has 30 calories of fat, or 4.5 fat calories per ounce. A whole can of undrained tuna packed in oil (soy oil, not even fish oil) has 297 calories of fat, or 45 fat calories per ounce.

Sausages and Lunchmeats

Sausages, frankfurters, and lunchmeats need to be regarded with suspicion. They can blow away your fat budget. Most are crammed with fat (in addition to being filled with dangerous additives and excessive amounts of sodium).

Don't Throw Your Kids to the Dogs

It is tempting to throw hot dogs into a pot of boiling water when your kids are crying for food—it's so quick and easy—but these cancer-risky packets of fat are poor choices for both you and your children. The poor eating habits established at these tender years as well as future dire health effects are not worth the convenience. In almost the same amount of time, you can coat skinless, boneless chicken breasts with barbecue sauce and broil them, steam some vegetables, and cook up some basmati rice (10 minutes) for a full, delicious, healthy, low-fat dinner.

Sausages and Lunchmeats	Amount	Fat Calories
Turkey frankfurter	1 frank (57 g)	70
Polska kielbasa	1 inch (28 g)	75
Chicken frankfurter	1 frank (56 g)	100
Cheese dog	1 frank (45 g)	120
Pepperoni	15 slices (28 g)	120
Beef frankfurter	1 frank (57 g)	150
Pork bratwurst	1 wurst (84 g)	198
Beef knockwurst	1 link (85 g)	210
Smoked link pork sausage	1 link (85 g)	230

Turkey and Chicken Franks: More Expensive Than You Think

Knowing that the American public associates chicken and turkey with low-fat, food manufacturers have created turkey and chicken hot dogs and sausage. Before you rush to buy, look at the labels. At 100 fat calories, a chicken hot dog is no buy. Turkey sausage may have 81 fat calories for a 3-ounce link.

Low-Fat Cold Cuts: Still a Poor Choice

If you use the cold cuts that have less fat (read the labels) and make your sandwiches less thick, you can fit cold cuts into your fat budget. But eat them with care. Although a hefty amount of fat has been removed, the excessive sodium, unhealthy preservatives, and high-fat taste remain.

This is true for low-fat and nonfat hot dogs too.

Sliced Turkey Breast: A Good Choice

At 2 to 8 fat calories per ounce, white-meat turkey that you buy at the deli counter is a good lunch choice. However, if you are buying packaged turkey breast, read the label. "Turkey" is not always synonymous with "low-fat."

Milk and Milk Products

Whole Milk: Not Wholesome

Most of us have grown up with the notion that whole milk is wholesome and pure and good for us. It's not. At 75 fat calories a glass (8 fl oz), whole milk is high-fat (and high-saturated fat, for that matter) and thus an unhealthy, fattening food. Drink 3 glasses a day (225 fat calories) and you have shot more than half of your fat budget. Don't give up milk—just choose lower-fat varieties.

2% Milk: High-Fat Milk

If moving directly from whole milk to skim makes you shudder, make the move slowly. First switch to 2% reduced fat milk. It tastes almost the same as whole. Whole milk contains about 3% fat.

Although labeled "reduced-fat," 2% is not a low-fat food. The "2%" refers to the fact that 2% of the *weight* of the milk is fat; the rest is water. At 45 fat calories per 8-ounce glass, 2% milk is far from low-fat. Get used to 2% milk, then switch to 1%. It tastes almost the same, but has 20 fat calories per glass.

Skim Milk: Work Your Way Down

Skim milk should be your goal. It has 0 fat calories per glass. Don't worry about calcium content. Skim milk has just as much calcium as whole milk, if not more.

Cream in Your Coffee

Keep a watchful eye on cream, for it is an insidious fat budget destroyer. Even innocent cream in your coffee can add up to large amounts of fat. One tablespoon of light table cream has 26 calories of fat. Four cups of coffee a day adds up to 104 fat calories, and for what? At 15 fat calories a tablespoon, half-and-half is better, but four cups of coffee quickly adds up to 60 fat calories.

If you are a dyed-in-the-wool creamaholic, cut the fat by drinking fewer cups of coffee. Better yet, be flexible, be adventuresome—try whole milk at 5 fat calories per tablespoon, 2% at 3, or skim milk at 0. Best yet, enjoy your coffee black.

Cream in Soups and Sauces

When you see the word cream, pay careful attention. Cream added to soups adds hundreds of fat calories. A cup of cream of mushroom soup has about 155 calories of fat; vichyssoise (creamed potato soup) has 210. When eating out, be sure to ask if the soup contains cream, and if it does, you may want to choose something else. You can budget it in, but if after a spoonful you find it is not worth the expense, push it away. Better choice: order broth or tomato-based soups.

Be wary of cream sauces. The creamy Alfredo sauce drowning your fettucine may cost you 873 fat calories. Even a half-cup of creamed chipped beef can cost you 100 fat calories. If every choice on the menu is covered with a cream sauce, ask that the sauce be served on the side. Try the dish sauceless. It may taste great without the sauce. If not, don't pour on the sauce. Use it sparingly. Measure out a tablespoon, spread it on, and taste the dish. Enough? More? Keep track of the amount you use. Spoonfuls quickly add up to cupfuls.

Whipped Cream: A Pricey Choice

Whipped cream adds a festive touch to ice cream sundaes, waffles, and hot chocolate. Enjoy a look, and then remove it. The perky dollop that floats on your cafe latte costs you 60 fat calories. The little cloud that nestles atop your ice cream sundae may cost more than 350 fat calories. Whipped cream splurges should be saved for extremely special occasions.

Cheese: Another Expensive Choice

The piece of cheese fits so nicely on the little cracker and tastes so good as it slides into your mouth. But it is rarely one little cracker and one slice of cheese. As you repeat this ritual over and over, talking, sipping a glass of wine, barely paying attention, you are consuming hundreds of fat calories. At 70 to 85 fat calories per ounce of cheese (of course the crackers contribute a stack of fat too), you have soon spent your fat budget for a day or two. Pay attention! You don't have to give cheese up completely, but you do need to watch the amount you eat. Buy a small quantity of your favorite as a rare treat. Eat it slowly. You will taste every bite.

Eggs: A Fat Packet

Eggs pack a lot of fat—50 fat calories in the yolk. Just the eggs in a four-egg omelet contain 200 fat calories. That's without the 100-plus fat calories added to cook them. To reduce the fat, ask for an omelet that has one egg and three egg whites. It won't be low-fat, but it will be a better choice. Egg substitutes are also an option. Ask that your fat-free omelet be cooked in a Teflon pan. If that isn't possible, find out the amount and what kind of fat is being used so you can figure out how much the cooking fat is costing you. If the price is too high, order something else.

Fats

Butter and Margarine: Spreads That Cause Spread

Of course everyone knows that butter is fattening. But how fattening? A tablespoon contains 100 fat calories. Think about that each time you prepare to slather butter over a piece of toast or drop it into a baked potato. Think about the assault on your fat budget when you eat your vegetables drowned in butter. One hundred fat calories for one little tablespoon.

Many people think margarine is lower in fat, but it isn't. It is a somewhat better choice because it is less saturated than butter (18 saturated-fat calories per tablespoon versus 65). Saturated fat contributes to raising blood cholesterol and thus risk for heart disease. However, it is now known that the trans fats in margarines behave like saturated fats in the body. So, although margarine has a heart-healthy reputation, it is just as fattening as butter, almost as heart-risky, and should be limited.

A tip: Always say, "Hold the butter!" when you order a sandwich. Sandwiches often come buttered no matter what the ingredients.

Olive Oil: The Most Heart-Healthy Fat

Olive oil contains mainly monounsaturated fat and little saturated or polyunsaturated fat. Extensive research has determined that olive oil lowers bad cholesterol (LDL) without lowering good cholesterol (HDL).

In addition, by preventing the oxidation of LDL remnants, olive oil helps prevent the first step of the atherosclerotic process. Having said all this, we still urge you to use caution in eating olive oil. One tablespoon of olive oil contains 119 fat calories! So, when choosing a fat, choose olive oil, but don't use a lot.

Mayonnaise: Pure Fat

One tablespoon of regular mayonnaise has 100 calories of fat. That explains why tuna salad, chicken salad, and shrimp salad sandwiches are so high in fat—they are swimming in mayonnaise. Think twice (or maybe three or four times) before you eat a meat salad sandwich (unless you make them yourself with nonfat mayonnaise). Make sure that your bread is mayonnaise-free. Use mustard instead and save yourself 100 fat calories.

Salad Dressings

A little girl interviewed on television was asked what her favorite vegetable was. She answered, "Salad dressing." What refreshing honesty! Salad dressing is the number one reason salad is so popular.

Salad dressing is a killer. One tablespoon of ranch dressing has about 85 fat calories, 1 tablespoon of creamy French about 70. But who eats 1 tablespoon? Or 2 (170 fat calories)? Or even 4 (340 fat calories)? Isn't it more like 8 (680 fat calories)?

Pasta

Many people complain that they are eating pasta but not losing weight. But which pasta dish are they eating? Lasagna (475 fat calories)? Spaghetti with meatballs (351 fat calories)? The sauces atop the pasta are the problem. Even one-quarter of a cup (one-quarter cup!) of Contadina's reduced-fat (reduced-fat!) pesto sauce has 170 fat calories.

For no strain on your fat budget, boil up your own pasta and cover it with a low-fat sauce. Sauté some tomatoes, lots of garlic, and a generous pinch of oregano in a teaspoon of olive oil, and within minutes you'll be enjoying a feast. You can also find commercial low-fat or nonfat tomato sauces in the grocery store. But remember, use sense. Eating a 16-ounce box of pasta will not make you fat, but your body will burn those 1,600 total calories instead of burning fat from your fat stores.

Frozen Meals

If you or your significant other are active members of the microwave age, we beg you to let your membership lapse. Take a few minutes and make your own food from scratch. It tastes much, much better, you can have more to eat, and it is much more nutritious. What's more, cooking is easy, fun, and creative. Express yourself.

A Box Is Not Dinner

If you want to change your ways slowly and are not quite ready to try cooking entrées, at least buy fresh vegetables to enhance your frozen dinners. Buy an inexpensive metal steamer in a kitchen store, department store, drug store, hardware store, or dime store. Place it in a saucepan with about an inch of water. Cut a vegetable—broccoli, carrots, zucchini, and so on—into bite-size pieces and put them on the steamer. Bring the water to a boil, cover the pot, and steam until tender. It takes only about 3 to 5 minutes to cook most vegetables. Bake a sweet potato or butternut squash. Boil up some rice. It's easy and well worth the effort. You need to eat delicious, nutritious foods to lose weight and enhance your health.

Nutrition Labels: You Gotta Read Them

If you do buy frozen dinners, learning how to read a label is essential for survival. The package may advertise a low-fat entrée such as fish, turkey, or chicken, but that is no guarantee the dinner is low-fat. The name may imply good health, but that is no guarantee that the contents are low in fat and healthy. For example, Healthy Choice's Country Breaded Chicken has 80 fat calories. This doesn't seem like such a healthy choice to us. Read the nutrition label to be safe.

Ruining a Good Thing

Hesto Presto Chango! See how the commercial food processors transform a low-fat chicken breast (13 fat calories) into a high-fat food.

Chicken	Fat Calories
Chicken breast without skin	13
Stouffer's Chicken Breast with Barbecue Sauce	210
Kid Cuisine Cosmic Chicken Nuggets	230
Banquet Fried Chicken Meal	240
Marie Callender's Chicken Pot Pie	880

Less Fat Means Less Food

In response to the public's desire to become thin, the food industry has reacted by creating hundreds of new low-fat products. A variety of truly low-fat dinners (fat calories ranging from 9 to 45) can be found in your grocery's freezer cases. Why aren't we applauding? The problem is that many low-fat dinners are low-fat because they contain so little meat (many contain about ½ to 1 ounce of meat). As a result, eating one dinner doesn't satisfy you. That is not to say that we recommend eating he-man portions of any meat. Eating modest amounts of meat is fine (and even healthy), but if consuming one low-fat dinner (45 fat calories) leaves you hungry for another (45 + 45 = 90 fat calories) and another (45 + 45 + 45 = 135) or leads you to binge on high-fat snacks to fill up your stomach and psyche, then low-fat frozen dinners are not a healthy choice.

Convenience-Store Foods

You stop at your local 7-Eleven and pick up a beef and bean burrito for lunch. You zap it in the office microwave, and in an instant your 240 calories of fat is ready. How convenient! As a bonus, you get to consume 90 saturated-fat calories too. Or try one of these microwave sandwiches if you want to blow your fat budget away. A set of little twin sausage sandwiches costs 210 fat calories, and a set of Chicken Chimichangas costs 200 fat calories. The Big 'Un is a humdinger at 440 fat calories. A Ham 'n Cheese Hot Pocket costs 220 fat calories; a Pepperoni Pizza Hot Pocket costs 260 fat calories.

The offerings at convenience stores are limited, but almost every one is a fat-budget destroyer. You will notice that almost every food is packaged for an individual to pick up and eat on the run. Chips, crackers, cookies, cakes, doughnuts, hot dogs, chili dogs—the package is small but the fat content is huge.

Even the few foods that don't contain a lot of fat—breakfast cereals, for instance, such as Frosted Flakes, Cocoa Frosted Flakes, Fruit Pebbles—are the poorest choices of that type of food. These cereals are high in empty sugar calories and artificial coloring and low in fiber and nutrition.

Convenience foods can be dangerous to your health.

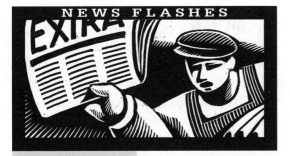

Milk Drinking Linked to Weight Loss

WEST LAFAYETTE, Ind.—Skim milk is relatively inexpensive, and according to a recent study, drinking it may help people to keep from gaining weight. In a study of 54 subjects, those who took in at least 1,000 milligrams of calcium a day (about 3 cups of skim milk) gained 6 to 7 fewer pounds over 2 years than those with low-calcium diets. Calcium probably prevents weight gain by increasing the breakdown of body fat and decreasing its formation, says Dorothy Teegarden, Ph.D., of Purdue University, the study author. "Calcium worked best when taken from dairy foods rather than through supplements or leafy greens," she says.

Size of Waist Could Be Connected to Risk for Colon Cancer

PITTSBURGH—Men with waists larger than 36 inches are twice as likely as thinner men to develop colon cancer. This was the finding of a 6-year study that monitored 5,849 people. "Having fat around your belly is associated with increased insulin levels, and that may encourage colon cancer to grow," explains the University of Pittsburgh's Robert Schoen, M.D., the study author. Since colon cancer kills about 23,000 men every year, that's another incentive for men to watch their diets and, if they're over 50, to undergo a colon cancer test at their annual physicals.

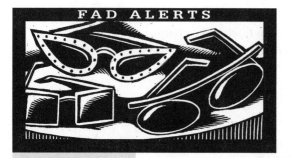

Products Sweetened with Fruit Juice

People who are trying to lose weight have no doubt noticed the many packages of cookies and drinks that advertise that they are sweetened with fruit juice. Many consumers assume that if the label says "naturally sweetened," the product must be healthier. This isn't so. "Sugar is sugar, whether it comes from corn syrup or fruit juice," says Leslie Bonci, R.D., director of the sports-medicine nutrition program at the University of Pittsburgh Medical Center. Juice-sweetened preserves or cookies have just as many calories as the regular kind, and no extra nutrients. So whether a customer chooses to eat these products should be a matter of taste, not health. And, as with any cookie, customers who are trying to lose weight should be careful not to overdo.

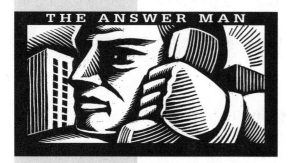

A Winning Combination?

My girlfriend is on a food-combining diet. She says certain foods aren't properly digested if you eat them in the same meal. Sounds like crap to me, but she's lost 12 pounds. Is there anything to this?
—D. A., Reno

Not really. Food-combining diets have gone in and out of style for years, but there's no scientific evidence to support the idea that eating certain combinations of foods improves digestion. "The human digestive system is well-equipped to digest foods in any combination," says Edith Howard Hogan, R.D., a spokeswoman for the American Dietetic Association. "Certain foods, such as beans and oatmeal, already contain both starch and protein, and your body digests them just fine," says Hogan.

So why do these diets lead to weight loss, at least in the short term? Because by separating meat and starches, you're forced to eliminate a lot of fattening foods (think cheeseburgers, foot-long subs, sausage pizza). "Eating this way is so restrictive that you end up eating less," says Hogan. But what makes food combining work initially can make it impossible to stick to. "And any eating program you can't stick with for the rest of your life is a waste of time," he says.

An Oil to Strike

What exactly is partially hydrogenated vegetable oil, and why does it seem to be in everything?
—K. B., Stowe, Mass.

It's a liquid vegetable oil that's been hardened through chemical processing so it's solid at room temperature, says Connie Diekman, R.D., spokeswoman for the American Dietetic Association. Food manufacturers love the stuff because it has a long shelf life, which is why it's in virtually all processed foods: packaged cookies and crackers, boxed macaroni and cheese, rice-and-sauce mixes, and other bomb-shelter fare.

Nutritionally speaking, hydrogenated oil is downright surly. It's high in trans fatty acids, a type of fat that's been shown to raise cholesterol levels. And like all other fats, hydrogenated oils will make you chubby and unhealthy if you eat them in large quantities. The FDA is concerned about the health effects of these oils, and by early next year will require manufacturers to list trans fatty acid content on nutrition facts labels. Until they do, scan food labels for partially hydrogenated oil. The closer it is to the top of the ingredient list, the more trans fats the food contains.

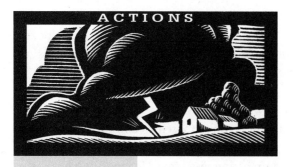

Wouldn't it be nice to lose weight and retire those relaxed-fit jeans? And no one needs to tell you that a beer belly isn't exactly a babe magnet. But if you need greater motivation than this to lose weight and get fit, consider the following:

- Physically fit men are 53 percent less likely to die a premature death than unfit men.
- Fit men are four times less likely to die from cancer than the unfit.
- Fit people are eight times less likely to die from cardiovascular disease than those who are unfit.

So how do you drop those extra pounds and get fit? Read on.

1. Sweat to the sitcoms. Convinced you don't have time to exercise? A sad but true fact: The average 35- to 54-year-old guy watches 27 hours of television a week, or roughly 4 hours a day. If you spent just half that time doing calisthenics while you watched, you'd burn about 825 calories—more than the burn you'd get in an hour of cross-country skiing at a moderate pace.

2. Think milk instead of eggs in the morning. To end those morning cravings for Egg McMuffins, drink a glass of skim milk as soon as you wake up. Some quick protein before you even step into the shower will energize you and end those hankerings for high-fat foods.

3. Learn the lingo. Food packages are full of fancy buzzwords, but it's easy to be misled if you don't know what they mean. Consider this your decoder ring:

- Regular: Greater than 3 grams of fat per serving
- Reduced-fat: 25 percent less fat than regular
- Light or lite: 50 percent less fat than regular
- Low-fat: No more than 3 grams of fat per serving
- Nonfat or fat-free: Less than 0.5 gram of fat per serving

4. For a better bike workout, count. Beginning riders have a tendency to ride in high gears, which gets tiresome quickly to both your legs and your lungs. Instead, stay in lower, easy-to-push gears and keep the pedals revolving quickly.

Try to always keep your pedal speed (the cadence) at 80 revolutions per minute or higher (serious bikers often sustain more than 100 revolutions per minute). Once you get your pedal speed established, use your gears to maintain that rate as grades or terrain change. The goal is to get your pedals to turn at roughly the same rate—a little slower going uphill, a little faster on the descents. Theoretically, it's possible to count, shift, and ride. But you can spare yourself the hassle by purchasing a cyclometer that also measures cadence.

5. **To keep off extra pounds, think zinc.** Researchers from Wayne State University in Detroit and the University of Michigan in Ann Arbor looked at the link between zinc and serum leptin—a hormone that helps regulate body fat by telling your brain when you've had enough to eat. An increase in zinc consumption makes leptin levels rise, causing your body to build muscle instead of fat. Grill a lean hamburger and eat it on a whole wheat bun for a high-zinc meal.

6. **Put a lid on it.** You can dramatically reduce the amount of oil (read: fat) needed to pan-fry foods simply by keeping the lid on the pot. The lid catches and returns moisture that would normally escape, thus preventing the need for more oil.

7. **Think like a guy at the bar.** You shouldn't need a reason to stay away from girl drinks, but here's one anyway: A piña colada provides 392 calories and 10 grams of fat. A can of Bud has only 145 calories and no fat at all.

8. **Take two.** Do 2 minutes of pushups every morning. Sure, it's tough to exercise as soon as you roll out of bed, but you can burn off 21 calories a day. That adds up to 2½ pounds in a year.

9. **Fill 'er up.** You don't have to deprive yourself to lose weight. You simply have to know which foods will fill you up without a lot of calories. Become friends with foods that are high in fiber and water content, such as these:
- Low-fat (1%) or nonfat milk
- Broth-based soups, such as vegetable, chicken rice, or minestrone
- Raw vegetables dipped in reduced-fat dressing
- Berries, citrus fruits, and melons
- High-fiber cereal (at least 3 grams per serving) with 1% or nonfat milk
- Vegetable juice
- Nonfat frozen yogurt topped with fruit
- As much low-fat (less than 3 grams per serving) tuna salad, turkey, or ham as you want. Toss it around with nonfat mayo or lemon juice and some pepper and fresh vegetables

10. **Make a weaker brew.** Fruit juice is made from fruit, so it has to be low in calories, right? Think again. A 16-ounce bottle of cranberry-grape blend, for example, contains 340 calories. So dump half and store it, then refill the bottle with water. You'll barely notice the difference, and you'll cut half the calories.

11. **Take a sniff.** Studies have shown that once you start eating, smelling your food can make you stop eating sooner by satisfying you faster. So savor the bouquet instead of rushing like a running back through your dinner.

12. **Don't drop anchor for fast-food fish.** Sure, fish offers lots of health benefits. But not the kind of fish you get at the drive-thru. McDonald's Filet-o-Fish, for example, has 450 calories and 25 grams of fat, twice the calories and three times the fat of the basic burger.

13. **Stand straighter by crunching.** Doing exercises that target the midsection can help you get stronger and stand straighter. In that vein, you'll look fitter, like you've lost maybe 5 or 10 pounds. So work stomach crunches and sit-ups, where you lie on your back, knees bent, and slowly curl your upper torso until your shoulders leave the floor, into your exercise routine. These exercises are great for toughening the midriff and building a strong muscle base. Try doing three sets of 10 to 15 crunches per set. To give your muscles time to recover, allow a day of rest between workouts.

14. **Pick a pepper.** Eating spicy foods will make you eat more slowly, fill you up more quickly, and slightly increase your metabolism so you burn more calories—three strong reasons to put a sprinkle of cayenne on that chicken.

15. **Think small meals for a smaller stomach.** A study at St. Luke's-Roosevelt Hospital in New York found that obese people who were on an extremely restricted diet reported feeling fuller when tested after 4 weeks than when they were tested the first time. The researchers suspect that overeating increases the amount of food your stomach can hold, causing you to need to eat more to feel full. If you want to shrink your stomach, eat smaller meals for several weeks. And be prepared to endure some hunger pangs as your stomach becomes accustomed to less fodder.

16. **Have a tall one.** Order cocktails in a tall glass. If you're having a scotch and soda, order it in a tall glass and add more low-cal soda to dilute the high-calorie alcohol. It will go down smoother and leave less of an impression on your gut.

17. **Nosh on Newtons.** When you have a craving for a sweet snack, you may be craving more than just sugar. You might also have a hankering for a certain texture—the chewiness of a caramel, for example, or the creaminess of a chocolate mousse. To combine both sweetness and the right sensory experience, try fig bars. Some are fat-free, but even those that do have fat are healthier than their cousins over in the candy aisle.

18. **Go solo, Han.** The more people around the table, the more you tend to eat. Researchers at Georgia State University in Atlanta found that when you eat with one companion, your consumption rises by 28 percent. With two companions, you eat 41 percent more, and with six or more dinner partners, you eat a whopping 76 percent more food.

5

DISEASE-
PROOFING

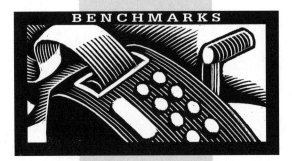

■ Number of Americans who are at least 100 years old: 62,000

■ Factor by which average air pollution levels inside a moving car on a highway in Los Angeles exceed those outside the vehicle: 10

■ Projected rank of heart disease and severe depression as the leading causes of death and disability in 2020: 1, 2

■ Percentage of deadly cardiovascular-related events that happen without warning: 33

■ Percentage change since 1930 in the annual U.S. death rate for all cancer : +11

■ Percentage change since 1930 in the U.S. death rate for all cancers except lung cancer: −20

■ Chance that an American without health insurance earns at least $50,000 per year: 1 in 4

■ Change since 1987 in a U.S. household's average annual spending on health insurance: +$323.28

■ Change since 1987 in a U.S. household's annual spending on medical services, supplies, and drugs : −$99.69

■ Percentage of American *ER* viewers who say they learn important health care information from the television show: 53

■ Factor by which "a cynical view" and an "aggressive" personality may increase arterial calcium deposits: 2

■ Chances that a sunscreen labeled SPF 30 provides an SPF below 30: 4 in 5

■ Percentage by which the incidence of skin cancer rises for every 1 percent decrease in the size of the ozone layer: 2

■ Number of times by which the size of the ozone hole over Antarctica now exceeds the size of the continental United States: 3

■ Estimated yearly amount the Pentagon spends on Viagra: $50,000,000

■ Number of yearly eye injuries caused by vacuum cleaners: 776

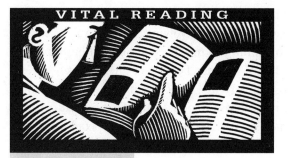

What's Making You Sick? Open Wide

Here's how five common diseases may be linked to
the bacteria in your mouth.

Farmers, cowboys, and other sensible men always examine a horse's mouth
before buying it. One good look can sum up the horse's health history and even
predict how long the old boy will live. A human mouth isn't much different. Just
look at John Elway.

"This horse test is based on the old 'focal-infection theory,' which says that
an oral infection affects the whole body," says Raul G. Caffesse, D.D.S., of the University of Texas-Houston Health Science Center. It was the excuse for lots of tooth
pulling until dentists abandoned the theory 40 years ago.

But the focal-infection theory is making a big comeback (minus the fun of
the extractions). And now it's supported by more than frontier hunches. In fact,
there's growing clinical evidence that small infections in your kisser may be a contributing factor to several diseases. Although the theories are still controversial,
dentists and other physicians think that the following five afflictions may be related to your mouth. That makes five excellent reasons to buy some floss—now.

Heart Attacks

When Robert J. Genco, D.D.S., Ph.D., of the University of Buffalo, studied
1,372 people at the Gila River Indian community in Arizona, he found that those
with gum disease had triple the risk of heart attacks over a 10-year period. He believes that oral bacteria (there are 350 different types in your mouth) enter your
bloodstream through small tears in your gums. The bacteria, Dr. Genco suggests,
may infect your liver and cause it to produce artery-clogging proteins, or they
may directly infect your heart arteries and somehow cause blockages. The exact
mode of attack is still a mystery, he says, but *Porphyromonas gingivalis* bacteria
have been found in fatty arterial blockages that cause heart failure.

You've probably heard that oral bacteria can be especially dangerous to people who have heart disease. If you have an ailment involving the heart valves, such as mitral valve prolapse or a heart murmur, you may need to take antibiotics before receiving dental treatment, says Mark V. Thomas, D.M.D., of the University of Kentucky College of Dentistry in Lexington. Dental work dislodges bacteria and nicks your gums, sending a rush of germs into your bloodstream. That can cause bacterial endocarditis, an often fatal infection that strikes about 20,000 people each year.

Strokes

Men with gum disease could be destined for drooling and Depends. University of Buffalo researchers surveyed the health histories of 9,982 people from 25 to 75 and found that the 35 percent with severe gum disease were twice as likely to have had a stroke. Oral bacteria may cause fatty accumulations in the carotid arteries in your neck, causing blockages, says John Marler, M.D., of the National Institute of Neurological Disorders and Stroke. These little logjams often break apart, float upstream, and lodge in your brain. And if a tiny chunk dams up a blood vessel, your dancing days are over.

Diabetes

When a person with diabetes is fighting a bacterial infection, insulin works less efficiently. That can raise his blood-sugar level, says Perry R. Klokkevold, D.D.S., of the UCLA School of Dentistry. If you're battling diabetes—and about one in 17 Americans is—a gum infection can make managing the disease much tougher. When University of Buffalo researchers examined 168 diabetics, they found that those with periodontitis (severe gum disease) had the most trouble controlling their blood sugar levels. Uncontrolled blood sugar levels are what eventually cause the kidney disease, heart disease, and blindness that plague people with diabetes.

Gum disease probably doesn't directly cause diabetes, says Dr. Klokkevold. "This is a relatively new field of research, but we know that having gum disease will worsen diabetes," says Christopher Saudek, M.D., a diabetes specialist at Johns Hopkins University in Baltimore, Maryland. "People with diabetes should be careful to keep their gums healthy." And if you have both a gum infection and a family history of diabetes, get checked for diabetes immediately.

Ulcers

This point is still controversial, but some evidence suggests that the *Helicobacter pylori* bacterium, which can cause stomach ulcers, resides in dental plaque, says Sherie Dowsett, D.D.S., of the Indiana University School of Dentistry. She and her colleagues found that among 242 study subjects, 210 of them carried the bacteria in their mouths. *H. pylori* may migrate down to your stomach and proceed to eat painful little holes, which is why we think every bottle of Pepto-Bismol should come with a free toothbrush.

Pneumonia

With every breath, your lungs suck down a stew of bacteria, including *Chlamydia pneumoniae* and *Pseudomonas aeruginosa*, two bugs that cause respiratory diseases. Careful readers will have guessed one source: the plaque buildup around your teeth. Your immune system usually destroys these invaders. But when your resistance is low, such as during an illness or after surgery, they can infect your lungs and cause bacterial pneumonia, says Dr. Caffesse. This infection kills about 83,000 people a year.

"Get your teeth cleaned before you have surgery," he advises. The day before surgery is best, but a week before is still helpful. And bug your parents to floss daily and visit the dentist every 6 months; they're much more vulnerable to pneumonia than you are, young man.

The Six-Point Body Inspection Plan

You get your car inspected on a regular basis. Now you can do the same for your body.

Every catastrophe has its warning signs. Your car has a "check engine" light, the pipes in your basement rust long before they burst open, and your smoke detector beeps at you before its battery completely runs down.

But warning signs have their flaws, especially when it comes to your body. Sometimes they come too late. Sometimes they come disguised as heartburn. And sometimes you simply ignore them, covering problems over with duct tape rather than popping the hood for a closer look. Before long, there's permanent damage.

The way we see it, you've got two choices. Hire a staff of overpaid government engineers to monitor your body's systems from behind a bank of computers, or learn the basics yourself. It's not hard. Do a little maintenance here and there, and you'll find that most of the body's major systems are built for the long haul. Form a few healthy habits, learn a couple of mechanical skills, and run some regular self-checks, and you'll help ensure that your most critical systems are primed for as long a mission as you are.

Your Skeletal System

Without its structural 2-by-4s, your body would be no more than an amoebic blob. More than 96 million doctor's visits a year are the result of broken bones, sore joints, pulled muscles, and other musculoskeletal ailments.

How it's most likely to break down:

- Osteoporosis. Men over the age of 50 are at least 10 times as likely to suffer an osteoporotic fracture as they are to develop prostate cancer. Without some intervention, you could lose an average of 1 percent of your bone mass each year starting at around age 40.
- Arthritis. Fourteen million American men—that's roughly 10 percent of us—have arthritis.
- Fractures. The average guy will suffer two broken bones over the course of his life. For men between the ages of 18 and 44, the ankle is the spot to watch out for—one-quarter of all fractures in that age group occur there.

System check: Walk 3 miles at a brisk pace. If you finish in under 45 minutes without pain, swelling, or stiffness in your joints, your bones and joints are doing their job.

Your maintenance plan should include the following.

Stretch your workout. The best exercises for maintaining healthy joints are weight-bearing exercises, such as running. Recent studies have found no evidence that normal joints (those that have never been injured) are damaged by long-distance running. But be sure to stretch first. "It's critical to keep muscles from tightening up and causing tendon problems," says Scott B. Scutchfield, M.D., clinical professor of orthopedics at the University of Kentucky in Lexington.

Come down easy. Nearly 645,000 people injured themselves playing basketball in 1997, more than in any other sport. Men who have injured a joint are more likely to develop arthritis in that joint. "Joints work because they have two perfectly smooth surfaces that cycle against each other. But if injury causes an irregularity in one of those surfaces, then the constant movement wears it down like sandpaper," says Dr. Scutchfield. Before long, it hurts to move.

To make basketball safer on joints, protect vulnerable areas—your ankles, hamstrings, and lower back—with braces and compression shorts. Avoid sharp cuts, which are hard on your knees, in favor of wide turns that take three or more steps. And always jump and land with both feet, keeping them shoulder-width apart, to reduce the risk of twisting an ankle.

If you've been injured, consider trading in that backboard for a kickboard. Swimming is one of the best exercises for sore or previously injured joints because it's low-impact (there's no pavement to pound) and it makes all the joints in your body work together in a smooth, controlled way.

Get milk. Many men don't take in the recommended 1,000 milligrams a day of calcium, even though it could prevent as many as half of all osteoporotic fractures. You can get 1,000 milligrams in three glasses of milk or 3 cups of yogurt a day. (Men over 50 need 1,200 mg.) Or take a calcium supplement, and be sure you also get enough vitamin D, which is critical to your bones' absorption of calcium. One way to do that is to spend a few minutes out in the sunlight every day.

Respiratory System

By the time you hit 80, you will have taken around 700 million breaths. But your lungs are more than simply a breathing apparatus; they're also the battlefield where intruders are fought off. "The lungs serve as a barrier to threats from the outside environment," says Alfred Munzer, M.D., codirector of pulmonary medicine at Washington Adventist Hospital in Takoma Park, Maryland.

How it's most likely to break down:

- Asthma. There's been a 61 percent increase in the asthma rate since 1982. About 14.6 million Americans have it, and nearly 6,000 of them die of it each year.
- Pneumonia. More than 30 different bacterial, viral, chemical, and fungal intruders are known to attack the lungs. If successful, they cause air sacs to fill with fluid, slowly choking off your supply of oxygen. Thanks to antibiotics, this hasn't been the leading cause of death in the United States since 1936— it has been bumped to number six.
- Lung cancer. More than 90,000 men will die of lung cancer this year; nine out of 10 of them will be smokers.

System check: Hold a lit candle 6 inches from your face, open your mouth wide, and take a deep breath. Try to blow out the candle without pursing your lips. If you can extinguish the flame, your lungs are functioning within normal ranges, says Barry Make, M.D., director of the emphysema center at National Jewish Medical and Research Center in Denver.

Your maintenance plan should include the following.

Watch what you breathe. Pay attention to those pollution indexes the weather guys are always yammering about. If the Pollutant Standards Index tops 100, move your workout inside. "When you exercise, you take about 10 times more air into your lungs than you do at rest, so working out in dirty air increases your exposure to pollutants tenfold," explains Dr. Munzer. That can make you more susceptible to respiratory infection.

Break out the vacuum cleaner. Many researchers believe that allergens are behind the alarming increase in asthma rates. "For that reason, it's important to reduce your exposure to pollen, dust mites, cockroaches, and other common allergens," says Dr. Munzer. That means staying indoors, with the air-conditioning on, as much as possible during pollen or ryegrass season (the dates will depend on where you live); dusting and vacuuming regularly; and taking a firm stance against roaches. And open the windows for a few hours now and then to help keep indoor pollutants down.

Get your flu shot. A British study of 445 people as young as 16 found that those who had received flu shots were 63 percent less likely to wind up in the hospital with any of a number of respiratory diseases, including bronchitis, pneumonia, and emphysema. Ten bucks, 5 minutes, and a pinprick in your arm seem like small prices to pay for lung insurance.

Cardiovascular System

Heart disease is still the single biggest man-killer in the United States. Lowering your risk isn't just about low-fat meals and exercise. Little things can make a difference, too.

How it's most likely to break down:

- Heart attack. About 1.1 million Americans have heart attacks each year; one-third don't survive them. In a typical attack, a blockage in a coronary artery cuts off the supply of oxygen and causes the death of heart tissue.
- Congestive heart failure. An additional 4.6 million Americans are cursed with hearts so weak that even modest physical exertion causes shortness of breath and exhaustion.

System check: Have your cholesterol checked at least every 5 years (every year if you need to bring it under control); and have your blood pressure checked every 2 years.

Also be alert for symptoms that could indicate heart trouble. Discomfort in the chest, especially after physical exertion, may be your first clue that something is going wrong. It can take the form of pressure, burning, or a squeezing sensation; may radiate into the arms; and is often accompanied by shortness of breath, light-headedness, fainting, sweating, or nausea. Also keep in mind that one in three heart-attack patients has no symptoms.

Your maintenance plan should include the following.

Don't look forward to Friday. The most common time to have a heart attack is first thing Monday morning. Mondays and the end of the workweek are also peak times for dangerous disturbances in heart rhythm. "It's not just the stress of going to work that's a trigger, it's the stress of a change in routine," says Mehmet

Oz, M.D., associate professor of cardiac surgery at Columbia University, and author of *Healing from the Heart*. In other words, putting all your energy into your work, or trying to cram all your relaxing into just 2 days a week, could be a dangerous practice.

But what's more important to your heart than stress itself is how you respond to it. "Responding angrily or bitterly—to the point where your heart rate and blood pressure go up—is far worse than simply being frustrated," says Dr. Oz. Learn to control your reaction, and your heart is less likely to self-destruct.

Snack on nuts, not chips. A 12-year study of more than 22,000 men found that those who ate a lot of nuts were less likely to die of heart disease. And a separate study of nearly 800 French people found that walnuts are particularly good. Subjects who consumed a lot of walnuts (and walnut oil) had higher levels of heart-healthy HDL ("good") cholesterol in the bloodstream. "I'm a nut addict," Dr. Oz told us. "That doesn't mean they're for everybody, but in moderation they're certainly healthier than most snack foods."

Nervous System

According to a study from Boston University, the average 65-year-old man has an 11 percent chance of losing a chunk of his brain capacity if he lives at least 20 years more.

How it's most likely to break down:
- Alzheimer's. If you make it to 85, there's a chance you won't remember a thing. Nearly 50 percent of people 85 or older have this degenerative brain disease to some degree.
- Stroke. Stroke occurs when there's a rupture or blockage of one of the arteries feeding the brain. It's the equivalent of having a heart attack, and it's the number-three killer of Americans and the number-one cause of serious disability.
- Injury. Of course, growing old isn't the only way to lose your nervous system. You can also physically damage it—something that more than a million Americans do each year. (FYI, 8 out of 10 spinal cord injuries occur in men.)

System check: It's tough to spot your own troubles in this system, because it's easy to dismiss some of the key symptoms, such as headache, dizziness, weakness, or forgetfulness. The only way to tell whether the cause is neurological is to see your doctor.

Your maintenance plan should include the following.

Think hard. People with higher levels of education, who are likely to have challenged their brains more throughout life, tend to get Alzheimer's disease later than those who leave school earlier. "I don't know whether that's a good reason to go on for a graduate degree if you don't want one, but it does suggest that using your brain may help prevent dementia," says Robert B. Daroff, M.D., professor of neurology at University Hospitals of Cleveland. Do a puzzle, learn the Gaelic alphabet, or at least switch from ESPN to the History Channel every once in a while. Just keep those neurons firing.

Have a glass of wine. A recent 16-year Danish study of more than 13,000 people found that those who drank one to six glasses of wine per week had a 34 percent lower risk of stroke than those who rarely drank. "After Alzheimer's disease, it's vascular dementia—essentially small, asymptomatic strokes that cumulatively cause brain damage—that's the most common cause of cognitive impairment," says Dr. Daroff.

Get your vitamins. Vitamins E and C have been linked to decreased rates of Alzheimer's disease, and vitamins B_6, B_{12}, and folate are believed to fight vascular diseases that can interfere with the brain's blood supply. Dr. Daroff recommends 1,000 IU of E, 1,000 mg of C, and a B-complex multivitamin every day.

Don't drink and dive. Two-thirds of all sports-related spinal-cord injuries come from diving into pools. Eighty-seven percent occur in backyard pools, 46 percent occur during parties, and almost half involve alcohol. Never dive into water less than 8 feet deep, and stay out altogether if you've been drinking.

Digestive System

This may not seem like a critical system to everyone, but don't ignore it. Its workings can go horribly wrong.

How it's most likely to break down:

- Colorectal cancer. This year 57,000 Americans will die of colorectal cancer, one of the most preventable and curable cancers if it's caught early.
- Heartburn. This seems innocuous enough, but it actually causes patients more emotional distress than diabetes or high blood pressure, according to a recent study.

System check: This one's pretty simple. "A change in bowel habits is the most important sign to look out for," says Michael Wolfe, M.D., chief of gastroenterology at Boston University. If you suddenly get constipation or diarrhea without a change in your diet, something could be wrong.

Your maintenance plan should include the following.

Keep things moist. "The main reason people become constipated is that they're dehydrated," says Dr. Wolfe. Hard stools can increase the pressure in your colon, and in some cases they can cause part of it to actually "blow out," painfully poking through surrounding muscle. So rehydrate yourself: Drink more water. Eating more fiber (from such sources as vegetables, unpeeled fruit, and whole grains) can also help soften stools.

Squash heartburn. If you suffer heartburn more than twice a week, you could have bigger problems. Chronic heartburn can damage the lining of the esophagus, it can cause esophageal cancer (one of the fastest-growing types of cancer in Western countries), and it has been linked to asthma. The best remedy is a combination of an antacid (such as Mylanta or Tums) and an H_2-blocker (such as Pepcid AC). "The antacid works immediately to neutralize existing acid, and as it wears off, the H_2-blocker kicks in to prevent further acid buildup," explains Dr. Wolfe.

Take an aspirin a day. It isn't just for heart attacks. It may also reduce your risk of colon cancer by as much as 60 percent. "I recommend that everyone over age 40 talk to his doctor about supplementing with an 81 milligram baby-aspirin tablet daily," says Dr. Wolfe. And if you're over 50, it's time to talk to your doctor about a colonoscopy, the only surefire way to pick up colon cancer in its earliest, most treatable stages.

Immune System

The immune system isn't just your first line of defense against viral and bacterial invaders; it also plays a major role in battling cancer cells and even the inflammatory processes that lead to heart disease.

How it's most likely to break down:

"It's a fact of life that as we grow older, the immune system works less efficiently, leaving us more open to infections and disease processes," says Marianne Frieri, M.D., Ph.D., an immunologist and associate professor of medicine at State University of New York in Stony Brook. The immune system can also work too well. Allergies and arthritis are two common results of an overactive or misdirected immune system.

System check: If you're functioning, so is your immune system. But more than six respiratory, sinus, or ear infections a year mean that something may be wrong. Ask your doctor for a white blood cell count. It can tell whether your soldiers are holding their own on the front lines.

Your maintenance plan should include the following.

Become an extrovert. If you laugh a lot or have a wide social network—you frequently attend cultural events (monster truck shows don't count), see a lot of your family, or practice any sort of religion—you're statistically less likely to become sick. The connection is stress, according to Dr. Frieri. "Stress causes a release of brain chemicals that actually depress the immune system. But laughter, friendship, a belief system, all those things work to combat stress, and they've all been linked to stronger immune function."

Get the right amount of sex. A recent study from Wilkes University in Wilkes-Barre, Pennsylvania, shows that sex can also strengthen immunity. Of 111 men and women quizzed on their sexual habits, those who reported having sex once or twice a week had levels of immunoglobulin A antibodies (immune-system cells that form the body's first line of defense against intruders) that were one-third higher than those of either their less active or more active counterparts.

Go easy on bacteria. Doctors prescribe antibiotics to an estimated 51 percent of all patients who walk in with the sniffles. The problem is that taking antibiotics could unnecessarily suppress your immune system, making you more likely to develop resistant bacteria or to become sick in the future. "Unless your cold has progressed to a bacterial infection like bronchitis or pneumonia, antibiotics aren't indicated," says Dr. Frieri. Tell your doctor you'd prefer not to take them unless it's absolutely necessary.

And go easy on that gold-colored antibacterial hand soap. A recent study from Tufts University found that an active ingredient in antibacterial soap, triclosan, can alter the genetic makeup of the *E. coli* bacterium, producing resistant strains.

Germs, Germs, Everywhere

Bacteria are lurking everywhere, but most are harmless. Here's a guide to the places and objects you needn't fear—and those you should avoid.

What's more likely to make you sick: kissing your faithful mutt on the lips or licking the bottom of your shoe?

We'll give you a hint: There's a reason your dog's breath stinks.

Germs—the all-encompassing word we use for bacteria, viruses, fungi, and protozoa—cling like barnacles to almost every surface on the planet. Millions of single-cell bacteria are on your hands right now, and millions more are squirming around in your intestinal tract, breaking down the pork chops you had for lunch.

You have almost a pound of bacteria in your body. Eventually they'll even serve as your cleanup crew: When you die, they'll eat you.

Here's the problem: Whether we're talking about germs on our shoes or on Scruffy's tongue, most of us have little idea of which ones are good and which ones make us sick. We live in peace with roughly 99 percent of these microbes; only a scant few, such as the rhinovirus and certain strains of *E. coli*, can get nasty. Even then, in most cases the miserable symptoms you feel aren't caused by the germs themselves but by your immune system. Since white blood cells can't distinguish a cold virus from Ebola, they attack every uninvited guest with a variety of chemicals, including cytokines, which are molecules that act as virus-killing grenades. The blitzkrieg can give you aches, nausea, and fever.

Though the occasional infection makes you feel like hell, this daily microbe bombardment actually keeps you healthy, says Michael Norgard, Ph.D., microbiologist at the University of Texas Southwestern Medical Center in Dallas. It forces you to accumulate antibodies and keeps your immune system tough and alert, he says. Without this strengthening effect, called antigenic stimulation, your immune system would grow lazy.

The trick to staying healthy, Dr. Norgard says, is to parcel out your paranoia properly. Avoid the germs and transmission routes that really can make you sick, and let the local TV news worry about the inconsequential risks. To help you do that, we asked microbiologists to rank the germ-harboring potential of the following 29 everyday objects and places. Here's where the dangerous germs lurk, and where they don't.

Germs That Aren't Worth Worrying About

You might think these are brimming with disease-causing germs, but they're not.

Mold-covered coffee mug. Even if you take a swig of week-old coffee covered with aspergillus (the familiar green fuzz), there's little chance it will do you any harm. Just rinse your work mug with hot water.

Laundromat washing machine. The trace of *E. coli* from the last guy's BVDs won't survive bleach, so wash your whites first. But even if you use cold water and no bleach, 20 minutes in a hot dryer will kill the bugs. Try not to take home anyone else's underwear. Unless it fits, of course.

Bottom of your shoe. Unless you've been wading through the local dump, you're safe. Common soil bacteria tend to be harmless, says William Perreault, Ph.D., a biologist at Lawrence University in Appleton, Wisconsin.

A bachelor's kitchen. The next time some woman freaks out over your dirty stove, tell her that tests have found that a single man's kitchen is much cleaner than a single woman's. "Bachelors don't clean often, so they don't contaminate things with a dirty dishrag," explains Charles Gerba, Ph.D., a microbiologist at the University of Arizona in Tucson. There is virtue in lethargy!

Money. Even if the subway clerk has more dirt under his fingernails than you'd find in Charlie Sheen's diary, the coins he hands you are probably clean. Metal coins and paper bills are generally too dry to support bacteria, says Dr. Norgard.

Urine on the toilet seat. Although it's disgusting, urine is nearly sterile and won't harbor many germs, even hours later.

Gym bench. The salt in sweat inhibits the growth of most bacteria. But wipe it off for the next guy anyway. It's only polite.

Hotel bed. Bed linens are generally too dry to harbor dangerous bacteria, says Ted Eickhoff, M.D., of the University of Colorado Health Sciences Center in Denver. Sleeping atop traces of dried semen and other substances may be revolting, but you have a better chance of getting sick from the free breakfast buffet in the lobby.

Biological Long Shots

These things could make you sick, but it's not likely.

Your dog. Some dogs are coprophagous, says Dr. Gerba. That means they eat feces. When Scruffy laps your face, he can transmit *E. coli*, salmonella, or *Pasteurella multocida*, possibly giving you the trots. The risk that your mutt will make you sick is very small, but try to restrain yourself from kissing him full on the mouth, especially on the first date. And wash your hands after touching anything that's been in his jaws—including his tennis ball, his fetching stick, and the femur he uncovered in the neighbors' yard.

Your favorite table at the diner. The wet table in your corner booth hosts almost every lower life-form, and we're not even including Andy Dick fans. That's because the busboys usually wipe down tables with the same dirty rag. If you're lucky enough to sit at a freshly wiped booth, keep your silverware off the table surface, says Dr. Perreault.

The Communion chalice. If one of the parishioners sipping before you has streptococcus, you have a slight chance of picking up his sore throat, says Dr. Eickhoff. The alcohol in the wine kills most germs, so there's little worry here. But if you catch strep throat often, ask the priest or minister to dip the wafer in the wine.

Beer nuts at the bar. Many of the people who dig their fingers into the peanut bowl have come straight from the toilet and haven't washed up. There's only a tiny chance that nut-bowl bacteria will give you diarrhea, but those odds go up slightly if you take an antacid after dinner. Antacids reduce the stomach acids that kill bacteria.

Public swimming pool. Public pools often contain small amounts of cryptosporidium, chlorine-resistant protozoa that are usually spread by young children who accidentally soil their trunks. In the off chance that these bugs make it to your stomach, diarrhea could strike for up to a week afterward. So keep your mouth closed underwater. "As long as you don't swallow a lot of water, you're safe," says Dr. Eickhoff.

Fish tank. If you have even a tiny open cut on your hand, marine bacteria in the tank can cause a painful infection. When you reposition the laughing skeleton, wear a dishwashing glove. Use a net to retrieve the wedding ring.

Convenience-store coffee area. As at the diner, says Dr. Gerba, the filthy cleanup rag harbors diarrhea-causing microbes. Anything that touches your coffee or your mouth, such as the stirrer or the lid, shouldn't touch that countertop.

Minor Gambles

These aren't extremely common risks, but they're still worth avoiding.

Public pay phone. The local call may end up costing you $3, but the cold or flu is free. The receiver handle, mouthpiece, and buttons of any well-used pay phone can be loaded with influenza and rhinoviruses, warns Dr. Norgard. "I'd handle the phone with a handkerchief, and keep the mouthpiece a fair distance from my mouth," he advises.

Women's restroom. Women's restrooms generally contain twice as many harmful bugs as men's rooms do, says Dr. Gerba, probably because of discarded sanitary napkins and nonstop diaper-changing. Okay, you don't visit the ladies' room that often. But you're not the one we're worried about. Your toddler could pick up hepatitis A or salmonella in there. If there's a changing area in the men's room, use it.

Kitchen sponge. Sponges and dishrags are perfect homes for bacteria: They're constantly moist and full of tiny food particles. Using that sponge to clean the kitchen spreads filth everywhere, says Gerba. Disinfect your sponge each night by soaking it in a cup of water mixed with a few teaspoons of bleach.

Urinal handle, faucet, or doorknob in the men's room. These can often be tainted with fecal bacteria, including shigella, *E. coli*, and salmonella. If you somehow introduce those bacteria into your mouth within a few minutes (say, by touching the bread on your restaurant table), there's a slight chance they could cause diarrhea, says Dr. Eickhoff. After you wash your hands, make it a habit to use a paper towel to shut off the faucet and open the door.

Grandma's home-canned food. The government forces food manufacturers to heat-sterilize their products to kill clostridium, which causes botulism. Granny, however, is exempt from this law. Botulism is rare, but it's nothing to mess around with; it can be fatal. Persuade her not to can beans, which are most vulnerable to clostridium, and to stick to acidic foods such as tomatoes and pickles, which are naturally antibacterial. And always heat home-canned foods at 212°F—a full boil—for 10 minutes to kill any bacteria.

Definite Risks

The following germ carriers infect people every day.

Friendly greetings. Coughing and sneezing don't transmit cold and flu viruses well; you could be stuck in an elevator for hours with a sick coworker and never catch his cold. But shake his hand and rub your nose an hour later, and the next day you'll be a mucus factory. You can't easily (or politely) avoid handshakes, so wash your hands more frequently when a cold epidemic hits your office. But don't reject a proffered hand. Better to be polite and risk the sniffles than to be healthy and universally disliked.

Locker-room shower floor. The wet, well-traveled floor is a campground for the dermatophyte fungus that causes athlete's foot. And just thinking of all those discarded Band-Aids is enough to give you the willies. Wear rubber sandals in the shower. If your soap slides into a rarely cleaned corner, leave it for the janitor.

Hotel hot tub. As if the air jets tickling your butt weren't bad enough, you also have to worry about pseudomonas, which thrives in warm water and causes skin infections, particularly around hair follicles. Hot tubs can also harbor chlamydia, which can cause eye infections. (Your chances of getting a sexually transmitted disease through a hot tub, however, are almost nonexistent.) Foam is a sign of an unclean hot tub. Even if it looks clean, dunk a clear glass into the tub and inspect the water, advises Dr. Eickhoff. If it's cloudy or discolored, stay out. And don't drink it.

Preschool or day-care center. These places are chock-full of fecal bacteria. "If your kids are in day care, it's only a matter of time before they come home with diarrhea and stomachaches," says Dr. Eickhoff. If your kids have to be in day care, find a provider that separates the incontinent tykes from the older kids. Ask the staff to keep your kids out of the wading pool, if that's possible. Last, try to make sure that the staff members always wash their hands after changing a diaper.

Frogs, lizards, and turtles your child brings home. Because they live in slimy, stagnant ponds, frogs are covered with salmonella and fecal bacteria. When, inevitably, your little naturalist touches his mouth or his food, he may be giving himself a nasty bout of diarrhea. Have your kid scrub his hands after every outdoor excursion.

Your doctor's stethoscope and pen. Because doctors use stethoscopes to touch dozens of patients in a row and their pens sometimes become makeshift probes, these two items are usually crawling with infectious microbes. Good-naturedly ask your doctor, "When was the last time you cleaned that thing?" (Heck, he always asks you the same question; fair's fair.) If he doesn't take the hint, ask him to swab his stethoscope with alcohol before he begins your exam. And never borrow his pen.

A one-night stand. A condom can protect you from some things, but HPV (human papillomavirus) isn't one of them. That's why it's one of the most frequently spread STDs. Touching her genitals with any part of your body could transmit genital warts to you. These increase your chances of penile cancer. Vaccine trials are under way, but we've heard that line for years. For now, stop trying to pick up women at bars. Or at least stop succeeding.

A pure mountain stream. "Every stream is a beaver's latrine," says Dr. Gerba, who could make a living writing country-music lyrics. If you drink that sparkling, refreshing stuff, a protozoan parasite called giardia could lodge in your small intestine, causing nausea and severe diarrhea. No matter how clean the water seems, boil or filter it before you drink it. You can also purify it with chemical tablets.

Kitchen cutting board. If you don't properly disinfect your plastic or wood cutting board after slicing or chopping meat, the leftover salmonella or *E. coli* could make bedtime interesting for everyone. Use separate cutting boards for meat and vegetables, and rinse your board with diluted bleach after each use.

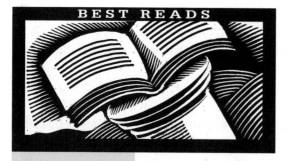

Memory Loss: Should You Worry?

Forgot the name of the new neighbor down the street? Misplaced your dry-cleaning receipt? What's going on—and should you worry that this memory loss is a sign of impending Alzheimer's disease? We all experience some memory loss as we age, points out Timothy Gower, author of Staying at the Top of Your Game: A Man's Guide to Peak Performance *(Avon Books). For most of us, though, this is nothing to worry about. As Harvard psychologist Daniel L. Schacter points out in the following excerpt, "Losing your keys is normal, but forgetting how to drive is not."*

After Michael Jordan nailed a buzzer-beater in the first game of the 1997 NBA Finals, a TV reporter asked him to list the most memorable game-winning baskets of his storied career. His Airness mentioned a few, but then a stymied expression came over his face. "That's the only two I can remember," he muttered. "I'm getting senile, I guess."

The irony was, well, unforgettable. Here was one of history's greatest athletes, a shade past his prime at 34, but still a rare physical specimen—worrying that his memory was turning mushy. And yet, one hears similar dark jokes all the time. Forget a phone number, struggle to put a name to a face, and out spill the cracks about obliterated brain cells and early-onset Alzheimer's disease.

First, the hard truth: memory does fade with age. Experts disagree when the great blur begins, but some believe that as early as twenty-five your ability to learn and recall new information begins to decline. The National Institute of Mental Health calls this tendency to forget more easily as we grow older "age-associated memory impairment," or AAMI. (In Jonathan Raban's travel memoir *Hunting Mister Heartbreak*, an Alabaman good ol' boy offers his own abbreviation: CRS disease, for "Cain't Remember Shit.") By age fifty, about 20 percent of us have developed a degree of forgetfulness that interferes with daily life; only one person in seven who reaches eighty does so with his or her memory intact.

Second, a little myth-busting. Simply forgetting things, even if you do so frequently—and even if your wife has sewn idiot strings to all your suits, so you'll never misplace your keys again—is not an early sign of Alzheimer's. "Losing your keys is normal," says Harvard psychologist Daniel L. Schacter, author of *Searching for Memory*, "but forgetting how to drive is not."

Age-related forgetfulness and the devastating amnesia characteristic of Alzheimer's are mediated by different mechanisms, he explains. The cause of Alzheimer's is still being studied, but researchers know that it's associated with a massive loss of neurons in the hippocampus, believed to be the center of memory and learning. Neuropsychologists once believed that people who become more forgetful, but who aren't demented, also suffer cell death in the hippocampus, only to a lesser degree. This posed a theoretical challenge to repairing a defective memory: brain cells don't regenerate, and you can't fix one that's dead and gone.

But in 1996, several studies using new brain-imaging techniques revealed that normal people suffer far less atrophy in the hippocampus than was previously assumed. The frontal lobes probably experience some cell loss, says Schacter, which seems to account for problems with so-called "source" memory—forgetting where you heard a joke, for instance. But the discovery that the hippocampus remains relatively intact buoyed the belief that malfunctioning memories can be repaired with medication.

Memory Meds

So far, though, few true memory aids have emerged. Alternative medicine proponents say extract of ginkgo biloba, the oldest known species of tree, enhances short-term memory by increasing blood flow to the brain. A *Journal of the American Medical Association* study showed that gingko supplements improved the memory of Alzheimer's patients, but proof that the stuff helps healthy people remember better is iffy.

Other researchers hold out hope for choline, a compound found in eggs and liver. The brain uses choline to make acetylcholine, a neurotransmitter responsible for relaying messages across synapses in the hippocampus. But choline supplements have failed to yield impressive memory improvements.

One of the most promising memory boosters to date has a peculiar history. Phosphatidylserine, or PS, is a compound that's highly concentrated in nerve cells. As we age, says clinical psychologist Thomas H. Crook, III, PS is displaced from brain cells by cholesterol, making them less fluid—a hardening of the neurons, if you will. He theorizes that the rigid membranes of aged brain cells are less receptive to impulses from other neurons, fouling up the retrieval of memories. PS supplements "fluidize" the membranes again, says Crook. In trials conducted at Crook's Psychologix test labs, in conjunction with researchers at

Stanford and Vanderbilt, subjects who took PS supplements dramatically improved their ability to match names to faces and remember phone numbers.

But PS had a little problem with PR: It was derived from cattle brains. Even those with the shortest of memories can recall the phrase "mad cow disease." However, a soybean version of PS hit the market in 1995. Crook recently completed trials which show that plant-based PS bolsters memory, too, with no threat of dire side effects. He recommends taking 300 milligrams daily for the first month, then shifting to a maintenance regimen of 100 milligrams each day. PS is available in most nutrition supply outlets, but not cheaply—a 100-milligram pill costs about a buck.

As for staving off Alzheimer's, a miracle drug is still not in sight. One study suggests that vitamin E delays the onset of Alzheimer's—but only if you take sixty-six times the recommended daily allowance. There is also some evidence that people who use a lot of nonsteroidal anti-inflammatory drugs, such as Advil, are protected, too. But doing so increases your risk for developing a peptic ulcer.

Drug-Free Memory Boosters

Doctors recommend other strategies for keeping the synapses sparking:

Stay mentally engaged. Groundbreaking research that compared well-educated elderly nuns with their unscholarly peers hints at the likelihood that intellectual curiosity keeps you from turning dotty in old age. Taking adult ed courses or doing the Jumble every day may not guarantee you'll stay dementia-free in old age—but giving your neurons a daily workout can't hurt.

Go for a jog. One study found that people who started aerobic exercise programs enriched their short-term memory, possibly by making more oxygen available to their brains. (Smoking tobacco can have the opposite effect.)

Eat food for better thought. Load up on citrus fruit, leafy greens, and fortified breakfast cereal; the B vitamins in those foods control levels of homocysteine, an amino acid that may damage veins, slowing blood flow to the brain.

Make a note. Harvard's Daniel L. Schacter tells concerned scatterbrains to carry around a "memory notebook," using it to write notes about things you need to remember. (Just don't forget to use it.) When making a note, be specific. Instead of just jotting down "Pete," write out "call Pete in accounting on Tues. re: payroll screwup."

Learn a new trick. If you have the time and patience to use them, mnemonic devices can help you retain important information. They work by associating things to be remembered with familiar images and ideas. Example: Say your new golf instructor's name is Jim Knowles. To remember it, picture him standing by a gym, atop a grassy knoll—only instead of aiming a rifle at the Kennedy motorcade, he's swinging a five iron. Bizarre, yes—but you won't forget it, will you?

There are, of course, many who say that middle-agers who complain of memory loss are simply distracted and neurotic. "Most of the people I hear complaining about memory problems are the 'worried well,'" says Paul Costa, chief of the Laboratory of Personality and Cognition at the National Institute on Aging.

Costa believes that significant memory decline usually doesn't begin among healthy people until they reach 60 or so. He's also found that people with the best memories at any age tend to be those who are simply confident in their ability to remember. If that's true, the next time you fret over a fuzzy memory, try this: forget about it.

The Fear of Growing Older

Even if you feel like you're still 25, age and ill health can have a shifty way of creeping up on you. A sudden unexplained pain in your chest or a strange-looking mole on your arm can leave you with a feeling of dread. In the following excerpt adapted from Dr. D's Handbook for Men Over 40: A Guide to Health, Fitness, Living, and Loving in the Prime of Your Life *(Chronimed Publishing), author Peter Dorsen, M.D., discusses two of the most common fears of men—heart disease and cancer. Read on to find out your* real *chances of getting these medical maladies—they're not as high as you might think—and, best of all, what you can do to prevent them.*

Aging confuses us. Some of us find it scary. We can easily fall prey to superstitions, unreasonable fears, or outright misconceptions. One response to our fear is to take the ostrich approach and ignore or deny the nasty subject of our aging as long as we can. But that approach may serve only to leave us more scared and perplexed by changes that will take place inevitably.

What are the things that concern us? You can probably come up with a list better than I can. But for now, do the following sound familiar?

1. Am I about to suddenly drop dead from a heart attack?
2. Do I already have cancer?
3. Why am I short of breath?
4. What's going wrong with my back?
5. Why do my joints hurt?
6. Have my arms become too short, or do I need glasses?
7. Is my hair thinning or merely migrating below my ears?
8. Is my hearing getting worse, or am I just not interested in what you're saying?

9. "I'm sorry, my dear. I swear this has never happened before." (Sure.)

Our first order of business, therefore, is to discuss some of these fears and put them into some kind of perspective. Just what are our risks of death, cancer, and physical impairments at this stage of our lives?

We can't alter the inescapable fact that you and all your buddies are aging. So it isn't just you. Aging brings changes—and yes, things will change. Such changes fall into three categories:

1. Changes that aren't really happening. (I'll call them superstitions about aging.)
2. Changes that can be reversed, such as poor physical shape, the condition of being overweight, and many sexual problems.
3. Changes that you have to learn to live with. (I'll call them the realities of aging.)

First, you have to separate the real from the imagined. In other words, you must clean out the first category and file what you find there in either category 2 or category 3. Sometimes this takes time. Sometimes we don't know what's real and what's imagined. And sometimes what's imagined becomes real, or vice versa. This testifies more to the weakness or the strength of our minds, depending on how that elusive faculty (the mind) is employed. But this discussion moves into another realm to be discussed in later chapters (deterioration of the mind), so right here, let's just keep this simple: Essentially, try to eliminate everything in the first category. What's left are the real physical manifestations of aging, some of which are changeable, some of which are not.

Arrrrgggh! Thump! (Or: The Fear of Dropping Dead)

I begin, naturally enough, with a concern that creeps into the male mind with increasing frequency with age—the fear of sudden death.

Imagine this scenario: You feel a pain in your chest followed by more pain radiating down your arm. You figure it probably came from that fall you took on the tennis court or from shoveling all that snow in the driveway last night. After all, your muscle tone just isn't what it used to be.

But then your heart starts pounding. You wonder: Could this mean you have a real problem, or is the pain just making you nervous? Should you go to the doctor or wait, hopefully, for the pain to go away?

You could be one of those men who literally never go to the doctor. Is such a pattern learned? You remember the time when you were waiting with your mother in your doctor's waiting room replete with fish tank, funny smell, and overused magazines. Your throat hurt. Your ears ached.

Then this large, red-faced man wearing a white coat came brusquely in, a round mirror with a hole in the middle of it perched on his forehead, a rubber tubelike thing swinging from his neck. Before you even had a chance to be afraid, run, or grab for Mom, "Open your mouth," he said, and stuck a fat popsicle stick inside. "Say 'ahh,'" he added, confirming that he would not set a conversation record. All you really wanted to do was throw up. When he stuck this pointy thing inside your ear, you knew then and there he had been smoking his pipe. Did any of this make you feel any better?

The chest pain continues, and you tell yourself, It's just gas, right? Or a spasm of some sort. Certainly nothing serious. You rationalize that if you were really having a heart attack, you would have at least had some kind of warning. . . . Right? Isn't that the way it works?

We've reached the age at which all of us have a painful memory or two to jar us—an old college buddy who dropped dead out jogging. Who can forget reading about the late Nelson Rockefeller, who apparently died while having sex, or seeing an obituary for a guy only five years older than yourself who just plain old dropped dead. Now you remember your great uncle Sam, who collapsed on his 44th birthday and never came back. All this is enough to make us legitimately fearful, though too often not fearful enough to do anything about it. You think, "I'll see if it happens again, then I'll take action." It seemed as if in most of the ER cases during my years of medicine residency at "The John" (Johns Hopkins) and later at Hennepin County Medical Center in Minneapolis, I was trying to determine whether one or another 40-year-old was or wasn't truly having a heart attack.

Sudden death may possibly be more explainable once the facts are examined more closely. Here's the real picture of how much danger you're in at any given time. My hope is in fact to lessen your fear.

- Under 40: At this youthful age, your greatest danger of dying suddenly could come from a congenital abnormality such as an absent left coronary artery (one that doesn't extend all the way down your demanding left ventricle). This is med-speak for existing heart problems that are most likely hereditary; that is, from a birth defect. This is how basketball player Pete Maravich died.

- Over 40: If you're in this crowd, your risks begin to shift toward such factors as arteriosclerosis (arteriosclerotic plaques causing coronary artery narrowing) and away from such congenital malfunctions that could pose risks to the under-40 set. This is especially true if you happen to have certain risk factors such as parents with a family history of heart disease, or if you have high cholesterol, diabetes, hypertension, or if you've smoked in the past 10 years. (Note: That's four out of five you can stick in category 2—that is, risk factors you may have a chance of correcting.)

Changes of Heart

It's important to be aware of those changes that are inevitable. Your cardiac reserve (just how much your heart muscle has in reserve when you stress it physically) declines with age, but that does not necessarily affect cardiac fitness. That's a personal biological matter related more to whether you decide to exercise regularly. In fact, age does not adversely affect your heart's response to vigorous submaximal exercise if you have chosen to remain fit. Things are looking up, aren't they?

Today's message: If you're fit, there's no reason why you can't exercise vigorously. Even though you're getting older, exercise and a healthier lifestyle (decreasing your risk factors) should continue to be beneficial. Just take the appropriate precautions.

That's not to say that many of us haven't heard of guys our age dropping dead totally without warning or explanation. It happens. But it happens so seldom that it's statistically not significant (that is, the numbers don't lead to any meaningful conclusions). I'm still one of those curious optimists who read the obituaries every day. I'm one of those weirdos who also try to figure out why an adolescent or 30- or 40-year-old has made the papers. My point is that for the most part, there is no reason statistically for a 35-year-old to get some ink.

Generally, if you don't plan to exercise too hard, or are one of those lucky few who are risk-factor negative—low cholesterol, good EKG, all four grandparents alive and vigorous in their nineties, are not a smoker and don't have diabetes or some combination of these—just begin exercising slowly and try to train with the assistance of a certified exercise specialist.

Rumor has it that as we age, everything we have shrinks except our noses. What a bummer!

Take heart—literally! This is one vital organ that actually gets larger as you age. Such "adaptive hypertrophy" (larger growth) is sometimes for the good, as in the case of an athlete's heart, or sometimes for the bad, as in the case of someone who has congestive heart failure, a condition in which your heart may begin to enlarge as it fails.

Raymond Harris, M.D., of the Center for the Study of Aging in Albany, New York, explains that the size of your heart actually increases between the ages of 30 and 90, largely because of heavier fibrous tissue in the heart muscle and valves.

But your heart can be a perverse muscle. As it ages, it may actually be shrinking even while it expands—that is, gaining in physical size but losing the myocardial (heart) fibers that make for a vigorous, efficient heart squeeze. This means that the heart, though it may be enlarging, is not doing so by adding supple, efficient tissue. It may be maintaining output, but it's doing so at a price. Long range, if this goes on unaltered, you may have a losing situation.

What happens is that an enlarged heart can no longer pump blood efficiently, and dilated heart valves can no longer be as efficient in sending blood up and out through the aorta to your vital organs. Though it's a bit more complicated, essentially the heart continues to grow (hypertrophy) in order to compensate, thus creating a rather vicious cycle. It's getting bigger but unfortunately not more effective or better.

Through cardiac enlargement and increasing stroke volume, a compromised heart can actually maintain adequate cardiac output, a vital ingredient for maintaining blood pressure and perfusing vital organs such as the lungs, the liver, and the kidneys. In plain English, stretched or otherwise aged heart muscle can pump just as effectively and achieve the same results as a healthy heart, but it requires care and conditioning.

But there are other possible complications. Failure of the electrical conduction system of the heart can occur at the same time as deterioration of the fibrous tissue in your heart. Your heart valves can thicken or become more rigid. These are aging, or senescent, changes your heart is inevitably undergoing, They're why a robust Kirk Douglas, still very much in the prime of his life in his seventies, suddenly passed out from a conduction disorder. With a permanent pacemaker, Douglas was back on the track again. An octogenarian and retired eye surgeon I know keeps outliving his pacemakers. His wife's biggest problem is getting him in off the tractor or back from cross-country skiing or tennis near his summer home in the New York Catskills.

More Changes of Heart

Your doc hears a heart murmur and becomes concerned. What, you wonder, is this all about?

By the age of 40, you should already know that the term "heart murmur" is not very precise. It refers to a wide array of gurgles, sloshes, hiccups, and burps that a heart may make in the course of beating. Kids' hearts routinely engage in such behavior as they grow and change. These are so-called "functional" murmurs, which are not necessarily of the same significance size as the valve abnormality. Once they've been checked out and evaluated with an echocardiogram, there does not have to be any immediate concern.

In the case of a 40-year-old man, however, there are certain possibilities that should be considered. Calcium plaques deposited on your heart valves may well be the culprit if your doctor suddenly discovers a new heart murmur. Just how much circulatory compromise you experience or is demonstrated on the echo determines whether a particular murmur is significant. In extreme cases, medical and surgical intervention may be necessary.

Other parts of the body can play tricks on the heart. For example, as you age, receptors in your neck become less sensitive to lower levels of oxygen or higher levels of carbon dioxide in your blood. Normally the function of such receptors is to increase heart rate to compensate for either low oxygen or high carbon dioxide levels. There is a chance you will run lower oxygen levels or higher CO_2 levels, especially if you have been a smoker. These receptors switch from sensitivity to low O_2 to high CO_2 levels as you age.

Doctors expect diminishing maximal heart rates on the treadmill as you age. A good rule of thumb of what to expect for a maximum heart rate can be determined by subtracting your age from 220. If you're 25, your resulting maximum heart rate is 195. But if you're 45, that number decreases to 180. In other words, as you grow older your motor just can't rev up as high. Most doctors aim to "stress" you between 65 and 85 percent of your maximum heart rate, using the 220-minus-age formula. Factors such as arthritis, level of fitness, or even unconscious fears about the test itself can determine just how well you will perform on the treadmill.

Acute physical strain, stress, or irregular heartbeats (arrhythmia) can accelerate your heart rate as you age. A fast or irregularly beating heart not permitting adequate left ventricular filling during diastole could ultimately compromise the amount of oxygen available to the rest of your body. This means that insufficiently oxygenated blood could fill your ventricles before its journey to your brain or to your lungs. The outcome can all too often be worsening heart failure, further arrhythmias, and even sudden death. And that's pretty much where we began this discussion.

And Now for a Word of Encouragement

The old saying "What can go wrong will go wrong" fortunately does not apply to the heart. As I pointed out earlier in this chapter, by staying fit you can, for the most part, ward off that heart disease bogeyman. I have run into many men who, owing to their genetic background, should have died in their fifties from heart failure but are still going strong in their seventies. Just because the genes happen to fit doesn't mean you have to wear 'em!

The Big C

If we were all being honest with ourselves, we'd admit that of all the potential killers of men at midlife (AIDS aside), cancer is the one that scares us the most. Death from cancer is reputed to be long and painful, sometimes, it seems, made worse by our own efforts to save ourselves. And the whole thing seems so unfair. Unlike heart disease, which often hits people whose lifestyles have caused them to "deserve it," cancer attacks randomly.

Does it?

Not if we take a look at some of the numbers as we compare cancers, especially with other big killers. Lung cancer kills more than any other form of malignancy. Overall, it exceeds breast cancer as the most common cancer-related death for either gender. And it can be largely, though not exclusively, self-inflicted (by smoking).

But if we're talking about a pure terror quotient, we have to recognize the differences among cancers. Some cancers have high rates of occurrence, but not of mortality. Skin cancer is an example. It has the highest rate of occurrence but is way, way down the list as a killer.

So what cancers pose the greatest risks to the over-40 male? And just how great are the risks?

Lung cancer, as we just said, is first. Colon cancer is probably second (behind breast cancer in the general population, but second as a killer of males). Third is prostate cancer.

Pass the Cigarettes, Please

Lung cancer is justifiably famous as a self-inflicted disease. It's true that the most reliable way of getting it is to smoke. There are other risk factors, however, some environmentally caused and some not. Radon gas in the basement can give you lung cancer, as can secondhand smoke. Certain jobs that expose workers to toxic fumes are also dangerous. These are theoretically preventable. But there are also non-environmentally caused cases, too—you know, the kind that just don't seem fair. Comedian Andy Kaufman, who never smoked and lived, by all accounts, a pretty clean life, was one of the more famous victims of lung cancer.

Lung cancer is to be avoided. What shows up as a dark spot on an X-ray can grow and metastasize if not removed. The mortality rate, especially if the cancer is not discovered early, is very high.

Yet the risk of contracting lung cancer without exposure to such environmental causes (like smoking) is pretty low. So if you are 10 years out from quitting smoking, certainly check your house for radon, avoid secondhand smoke, and get a chest X-ray regularly; statistics show you ought to be able to dodge the lung cancer bullet.

The Case of the Bloody Stool

According to J. S. Billett and M. C. Castleden of the Department of Medicine for the Elderly, Leicester, England, the colon is the site of the second deadliest cancer and is the second most common site of all cancer after skin cancer. A malignancy in the colon can often start as a benign polyp but end with wild growth and tissue destruction—that's why your HMO should always be anxious to go mining for polyps after you turn 40.

Colon cancer also has a surprisingly dismal prognosis. Yet the gastrointestinal system is another of those areas where listening to your body counts. Surveillance is the only reason, really, to discuss the statistics for colorectal cancer. In 1984 this brand of potential death struck 130,000 Americans (odds of getting it: 1 in 2,000), killing 60,000 of them. Three-quarters of the cancers involved the distal end of the gastrointestinal tract, often within a finger's distance of the rectum. Additionally, three-quarters of colorectal cancers are within the reach of a relatively painless diagnostic test, flexible sigmoidoscopy, a procedure easily done in any doctor's office. The American College of Physicians recommends for men over 40 to include a "flex sig" in their physical exam, and, if they are over 40, three hemoccult slide samples of separate stool samples (the simplest test for hidden blood in bowel). This is another way of testing for colorectal cancer. Keep in mind that polyps with cancer in situ won't test positive for blood until frank blood or even obstruction develops.

One caveat: There are false positive tests for blood in stool. The rule is that anyone who has his stools tested for blood should eat a lot of roughage but no red meat or beets for three days before collecting the samples. Seven percent of all tumors detected by this testing are still readily operable. The dictum is "listen to your body." You should respond as calmly as you can but decisively to pain, bleeding, or unexplained weight loss.

There's no question what must be done if your physician first detects blood in your stool or subsequently polyps during a barium enema, an easy way to "run your bowel." If you have any polyps detected and removed by the sigmoidoscope or by colonoscopy, a fiber optic study that goes all the way to the appendix at the end of the colon, you should then have either an air-contrast barium enema or colonoscopy every 1 or 2 years. Keep in mind that for a colonoscopy, you will get drugs intravenously that not only eliminate any pain but leave you amnesiac. Such a deal. A major consideration with colorectal cancer is that the chances of surviving metastatic colon cancer are grim. You want to catch it early and, hopefully, eliminate it completely before it ever spreads. Although 20 percent undergo partial remission, there is unfortunately little prolongation of life.

Another test to monitor for colon cancer recurrence is based on the fact that Carcinoembryonic Antigen (CEA) is elevated in colon cancer. A simple blood test for CEA can be used to follow the course of resected colon cancer and to detect any recurrence 3 or 6 months after surgical excision.

So Why Does My Doctor Need to Do a Rectal Exam?

Prostate cancer, the number three killer, hits about 70,000 men a year (odds: 1 in 3,000) as the third leading cause of cancer death in men. Black men are at highest risk, a hint that high stress can contribute to the risks. Again, early detection is crucial because prognosis is closely linked to the stage at which the illness is diagnosed.

Watch for the warnings. Certain symptoms are very suspicious. These include frequent urination, incomplete emptying of the bladder, or even embarrassing overflow incontinence.

Men over 40 should be tested for prostate cancer at least once every two years; over 60, once a year. Who wants to end up like Frank Zappa anyway? His prostate cancer had already spread. Make sure your examiner gets a substantial feel of your prostate for any lumps and bumps. He or she should draw a "male pap" blood test (PSA—prostate specific antigen), preferably before the gland has been squeezed, aroused, or obstructed. In case you were wondering, recent sexual activity can produce a false elevation in the PSA. Until recently, some insurance companies have been reluctant to reimburse for this examination.

Data show that any type of prostate cancer with only a few so-called well-differentiated clusters will not increase the risk of death above that of the general population without cancer. But if the disease evolves to diffuse cancer at prostatectomy (stage A2), you definitely face a higher risk of relapse and death if the cancer is not treated.

Stage B, treated like stage A2, means a localized cancer is palpable on rectal examination, and you are a candidate for either surgery or irradiation. Radical prostatectomy, however, has a number of unpleasant complications, including impotence and retrograde or backward ejaculation, sometimes even with incontinence. Irradiation, therefore, may just be easier on your system. Men who have stages C and D prostate cancer, which means the cancer cells are spreading (metastasizing), are candidates for irradiation (for local control) or hormonal treatment (for painful metastatic bone pain, unfortunately all too common for those with prostate cancer).

Recent studies conducted at Harvard Medical School suggest a strong link between prostate cancer and eating fatty red meat. A diet high in red meat is said to increase the risk of prostate cancer by two or three times.

Other Cancers

There are plenty of other less common cancers to worry about, but fortunately, the odds of contracting any one of them are pretty low, though the odds increase as you age.

Stomach cancer, although reputedly on the wane in the United States, typically numbers 25,000 new cases a year. That's a 1 in 10,000 chance of getting it. Here's a cancer that may have significant environmental causes, including dietary exposure to nitrates common in cured meats such as bacon and sausage as well as other carcinogens. If you are unfortunate enough to learn you have it, the cancer is usually already in an advanced stage at the time of diagnosis. Small-cell carcinoma of the lung is another "bad actor" because at the time of diagnosis in the lung, the cancer has usually spread to the brain, bone, or liver.

Another of the baddies is pancreatic cancer. It comes by its grim reputation for good reason. Of the 25,000 people diagnosed with it in 1984—again, a 1 in 10,000 chance of getting it—95 percent were dead in 3 years. The 5-year survival rate is 1 percent. Like stomach cancer, pancreatic cancer is too often already incurable by the time it is diagnosed. It usually goes unnoticed until you feel some vague, yet frequently painful, deep abdominal discomfort. Then, by the time you find it, it has spread everywhere deep in the abdomen. Only 5 to 15 percent of patients who undergo surgery for pancreatic cancer are alive in 5 years.

One fact we tend to forget is that men also get breast cancer—not to be confused with benign male breast swelling called gynecomastia, growth in your breasts from drugs, hormones, or during adolescence. Breast cancer in men is rare as hen's teeth, but plenty fatal if missed. Make sure your doc does a 360-degree exam of both of your nipples, as well as a routine exam of your testicles and rectum.

Testicular cancer, particularly a "germ-cell" tumor of the testis, actually has a rather low incidence—2.3 cases per 100,000 persons. Testicular cancer, like colon rectal cancer, is another form of the disease with a marker that normalizes after a favorable clinical response, meaning it can be followed by a relatively simple lab test. Treatment is generally castration (partial, if only one side is affected) followed by irradiation of the deep lymph nodes in the abdomen.

Fortunately, a stage 1 nonseminal germ-cell tumor of the testes responds well to surgery alone—that is, castration with a radical inguinal lymph node dissection up into the abdomen. The good news is that combination chemotherapy is capable of inducing a remission in as many as 80 percent of the patients who have a disseminated form of this particular cancer.

No conversation about the Big C can be complete without mentioning melanoma—to many a particularly frightening form of skin cancer. Although skin cancer, per se, is the most common kind of cancer, what prevents it from also being the most common killer is that melanoma, the truly dangerous variety of skin cancer, is relatively uncommon. But melanoma is on the rise. Increased solar radiation, ultraviolet light to be exact (especially if you are one of those fair-skinned Scandinavian types), accounts for age-adjusted death rates for melanoma of four to five times what they were 30 years ago.

As is the case with many other cancers, genetic predisposition is a factor. Further, the depth of a tumor has a great deal to do with its prognosis. Tumors of more than 4 millimeters in depth and through the dermis carry an 80 percent risk of metastasis to beyond the nearby lymph nodes. If you have a red-blue gnarly growth on the back of your neck, your back, your arms, your leg, or anywhere, go somewhere to have the best doctor look at it and, if necessary, remove it. A technique as simple as a punch biopsy is least invasive yet can effectively provide the essential information between an appropriate full excision or terminal spread.

You can also get one of the several "liquid" tumors, the leukemias, all having their own course and prognosis. Keep in mind that I had my own practice for 11 years and never once found a new leukemia. There are also the "solid" cancers involving the lymphatic system, which, on a good day, strains your blood of impurities. These include lymphoma or Hodgkin's disease. Among these there's a wide difference in prognosis. For example, a lymphoma with very bizarre differentiated cells offers a bleak prognosis. But this type of malignancy, in the hands of a good oncologist, can respond very favorably.

Multiple myeloma is an affliction of the line of plasma cells that are involved with the immune system. They are virulent despite favorable innovations in chemotherapy and more radical methods such as bone marrow transplantation. Of significance is that multiple myeloma begins to have its greatest incidence (3 in 100,000) in middle-aged men. Median survival is from 1 to 4 years, depending on the amount of tumor mass at the time of initial diagnosis. These kind of numbers are one of the reasons I did not go into oncology.

Don't Panic

What can you do about the Big C?

1. Watch for the signs, some of which I have indicated above. If your family has a history of cancer, be particularly vigilant.

2. Don't be afraid to have an abnormality on or in your body checked out. It seems to be the natural tendency of men to seek medical treatment—or pursue wellness treatment—less frequently than they should or than women do. If something's not right, don't be macho and just ignore it.

3. Make sure you get a proper diagnosis. If you're not sure after visiting one health care professional, get a second opinion.

4. After you get all the facts about your particular problem and the recommended treatment, do what you're supposed to do and try to keep a good attitude. Believe it or not, keeping a positive attitude is one of the best medicines you can get.

Other than that, don't panic. Numbers don't lie, and they suggest that maybe you ought to worry a bit less about cancer after adequate surveillance and more about your cholesterol level—something you may actually be able to control.

When you read the numbers, also keep in mind that these statistics are not cumulative. Your risk of colon rectal cancer has nothing to do with your risk of cancer of the pancreas. In other words, you do not add your 1 in 2,000 chance to your 1 in 25,000, throw in a few other cancers, and come up with something like a 250 in 1,000 chance of dying of cancer in the next 6 months. Chances are that even in the unlikely event that you do get cancer, you're only going to get one kind. So your maximum risk is really only 1 in 2,000 for the most common type. No matter what.

So here's the kicker: After going through the litany of cancers you can get by breathing the air, drinking the water, or choosing the wrong parents or locality in which you live, the simple process of the narrowing of your heart vessels is by far a greater, but simultaneously more avoidable, killer. Five million Americans have coronary artery disease, making it—not cancer—the leading cause of death in males over 35 and in all persons over 45. Nearly all excess mortality in men is due to coronary artery disease. Despite overall downward trends in cardiac mortality, there is still an increase in the annual incidence of heart disease between the ages of 40 and 65. So much for truly understanding the significance of the numbers for cancer compared with heart disease. Heart disease is still a plenty big killer.

I'm not suggesting that you stop being careful about the quality of air or water you breathe or drink. By all means, reduce your cancer risk where and when you can, because the odds are that once you reach a ripe old age, if heart disease doesn't finally take its toll, cancer will.

So quit smoking. Above all, reduce any cardiac risk factors you can control because that may be the most significant way you have to decrease your risk of dying earlier than you need to.

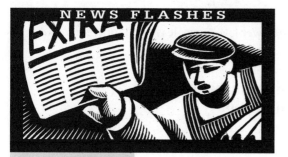

Drinking Apple Juice with Fast Food May Have Protective Effect

LOS ANGELES—Drinking apple juice may keep your cholesterol in check. Researchers at the University of California have determined that apple juice is able to reduce LDL (the bad kind) cholesterol oxidation—the process that causes cholesterol to break down into its artery-clogging form—by up to 34 percent. One reason for the juice's ability to attack LDL cholesterol is its high concentration of phenols, plant-based compounds that are also present in red wine. "Drinking apple juice with a fast-food meal may be enough to protect you against the fats you're eating," says Eric Gershwin, M.D., the study coauthor.

Zinc Intake Linked to Risk for Enlarged Prostate

CAMBRIDGE, Mass.—Taking extra zinc could increase your risk of developing an enlarged prostate. This was the finding Harvard researchers made when they conducted a 3-year study of 455 men. Specifically, the men who consumed more than 15 milligrams of zinc daily were three times more likely to have enlarged prostates than those who took less. Zinc may raise testosterone levels, which can spur prostate growth, speculates Dimitrios Trichopoulos, M.D., coauthor of the study. "Being a 60-year-old man myself, I would avoid any supplement containing zinc," he says. "It's easy to get your daily limit of 15 milligrams by eating lean meat."

Taking Multivitamins Could Prevent Periodontal Disease

BUFFALO—Brushing and flossing are still important, but taking a multivitamin could be one of the best ways to prevent periodontal disease. When researchers at SUNY Buffalo evaluated blood samples from 9,862 subjects, they found that those with the highest vitamin A and C levels had half the rate of gum disease of those subjects with the lowest levels. And high selenium levels were linked to a 13-fold reduction in cases of gum disease. "As the body fights invasion from bacteria in dental plaque, it produces free radicals that can damage gum tissue," says Sara G. Grossi, D.D.S., the lead study author. "Since antioxidants help protect against this damage, lower levels may leave you more susceptible to periodontal disease."

Potassium and Magnesium Intakes Possible Factors in Bone Density

MEDFORD, Mass.—In a 4-year study of 600 men, researchers at Tufts University found that men with the lowest potassium and magnesium intakes lost roughly four times more bone density in the hip than men with the highest. "Potassium and magnesium reduce acidity in the blood," explains Katherine Tucker, Ph.D., the study author. "When blood is acidic, minerals in the bone may leach out, resulting in osteoporosis." Spinach, oats, and wild rice contain both minerals.

Herbs Could Be Deadly Before Surgery

PARK RIDGE, Ill.—Herbal supplements can interact with anesthesia. The American Society of Anesthesiologists (ASA) has received reports linking ginseng to blood-pressure spikes and sudden heart-rate changes; St. John's wort to fever and high blood pressure; and Ginkgo biloba to impaired blood clotting in patients under anesthesia. "If you don't tell your doctors what you're taking, you may be jeopardizing your life," warns John B. Neeld Jr., M.D., ASA president. Stop taking all herbal supplements 2 weeks before your scheduled surgery.

New Screening Method for Lung Cancer Now Available

NEW YORK CITY—A new lung-cancer screening method could save more than 100,000 lives each year. Researchers have discovered that computed tomography (CT) screening detects lung cancer at an earlier stage than traditional X-rays do, potentially increasing 5-year survival rates from 15 percent to more than 80 percent. Claudia Henschke, M.D., Ph.D., of New York Presbyterian Hospital, the study author, recommends that smokers and ex-smokers visit a major medical center for yearly CT screenings.

Two Cups a Day Could Keep Gallstones Away

CAMBRIDGE, Mass.—According to a Harvard study, drinking coffee may guard against gallstones. Researchers polled 46,008 men over a 10-year period and found that those who drank 2 to 3 cups of coffee per day had a 40 percent lower risk of gallstones than men who didn't drink coffee. Since no risk reduction was associated with drinking decaffeinated coffee, it is thought that caffeine may stimulate the gallbladder to eliminate stone-forming cholesterol, says Michael Leitzmann, M.D., the lead study author.

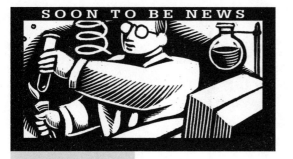

A Vaccine for Ulcers?

Don't stress out about getting an ulcer. A new vaccine may prevent the 22 million ulcer cases caused each year by the *Helicobacter pylori* bacterium. In one study, researchers gave 40 subjects either a pill containing inactive *H. pylori* or a placebo three times over the course of 28 days. Tests performed 6 months later showed that 100 percent of those given the vaccine had developed antibodies to *H. pylori*, while the placebo group had none.

Further studies to confirm these findings are being planned.

An Immunization to Prevent Tooth Decay?

A vaccine for cavities and plaque may be available within the next few years. When University of Alabama researchers gave the vaccine to mice, there was an 85 percent reduction in the bacteria that cause tooth decay and plaque. According to Suzanne Michalek, Ph.D., the lead researcher, the vaccine causes the salivary glands to produce antibodies against the bacteria. "We're hoping that in the future, immunizations will provide 100 percent protection against tooth decay," says Dr. Michalek.

Studies on humans are under way.

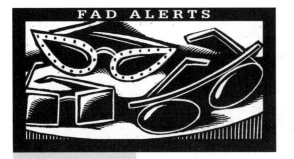

Alpha-Lipoic Acid

 Alpha-lipoic acid is found in small amounts in spinach, potatoes, and red meat. A bottle of 50 tablets of 50 to 100 milligrams can cost $12 to $20.

Over time, high blood sugar can damage nerves, causing pain and numbness in the hands and feet. Alpha-lipoic acid may promote blood flow to nerves to help repair this damage, says Phillip Low, M.D., a neurologist at the Mayo Clinic. It has no known side effects. In one study of 328 diabetics with nerve damage, those who took 600 milligrams of alpha-lipoic acid daily had fewer symptoms after 3 weeks than those who took a placebo.

If you have diabetes, talk to your doctor.

Selenium

Is selenium nature's answer to preventing prostate cancer? This mineral is found in seafood, liver, meat, and grains. The Recommended Dietary Allowance is 70 micrograms a day, but studies have suggested that taking 200 micrograms daily can reduce your risk of prostate cancer. A bottle of 200 pills (200 micrograms each) costs about $7.

Selenium may increase levels of the antioxidant glutathione peroxidase, which helps protect prostate cells. While studying selenium's effects on skin cancer rates, University of Arizona researchers found that men who took 200 micrograms of selenium had a 63 percent lower incidence of prostate cancer than those who didn't.

Until selenium is tested specifically as a prostate protector, it can't be determined for certain how effective the mineral is. "It's hard to know if the results on prostate cancer are real or a statistical fluke," says Peter Newburger, M.D., of the University of Massachusetts Medical School in Worcester.

That said, there's no known downside to taking the recommended dosage, especially if you have a family history of prostate cancer.

Isoflavone Pills

Countless studies suggest that soy can both help prevent prostate cancer and lower your cholesterol levels. Pill makers have tried to make soy more painless by extracting soy's nutritional value and putting it in capsule form. Thirty 60 milligram pills—about 10 days' worth—cost about $10.

Soy isoflavones—which are the main components in the pills—are estrogenlike substances. Since estrogen has been shown to have a protective effect on the prostate, the isoflavones may be the substance that's providing the benefit, according to Gregory L. Burke, M.D., of Wake Forest University in Winston-Salem, North Carolina.

Research does indicate that isoflavones and their weak estrogenic effect can help prevent prostate cancer. But isoflavone pills haven't shown the same beneficial effect on cholesterol levels as dietary soy has.

These supplements probably won't budge your cholesterol levels, and there is the rare chance—as with any estrogen-boosting substance—that they'll cause breast growth. So for now, it seems best to simply drink soy milk and hide some tofu in your chili.

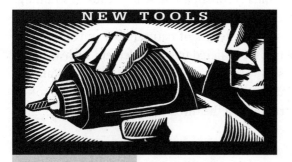

NEW TOOLS

A More Accurate Heart Test

MPI

According to a study published in the journal *Circulation*, a new test can detect heart problems that treadmill tests miss. Electrocardiograph readings were taken on 388 people taking a treadmill test. These readings were then followed by an MPI—a dye test used to find blood flow problems. The people with abnormal MPIs were eight times more likely than those with normal MPIs to have a heart attack or a serious blockage in the next 18 months. Sofia Chatziioannou, M.D., Ph.D., the study author, recommends that patients talk to their doctors about following up a treadmill test with an MPI.

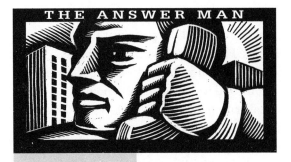

Staying Out of the Hot Seat

My two brothers and my parents suffer from hemorrhoids. Are they hereditary? Anything I can do to prevent them?

—C. O., Indianapolis

"Hemorrhoids do run in families, but they have less to do with genes than with lifestyle," says Janice Rafferty, M.D., a colorectal surgeon. "We learn our eating habits from our parents. And if you spend half an hour in the bathroom with the sports section just like Dad did, you're likely to develop hemorrhoids, too."

A common cause of hemorrhoids is constipation, which leads to straining, which causes veins to stretch beyond their normal size. Prevent constipation and you may escape your family curse. Include lots of natural fiber in your diet by eating fruits and vegetables, and take a powdered fiber supplement such as Metamucil every day. It's a safe and easy way to prevent constipation, says Dr. Rafferty. Finally, and most important, drink 8 to 12 glasses of water a day. Water will soften your stool and keep you from straining on the throne.

Multis and Meds

Is it okay to take my vitamins at the same time as my prescription medication?

—F. T., Woodbine, Ga.

It's generally okay to take all your pills in one gulp, says Arthur Jacknowitz, Pharm.D., of West Virginia University. But some combinations could be trouble. Taking high doses of vitamin C—500 milligrams or more—can neutralize tricyclic antidepressants, such as Elavil and Tofranil. (Prozac is in a different class of antidepressants; there are no studies that suggest it's affected by vitamins.) And if you take the anticoagulant Coumadin for high blood pressure, don't take vitamin E, which is also an anticoagulant. The combination can cause severe bleeding in some people. For more details on specific drug interactions, talk to your pharmacist.

Ask a Doc What's Up

I'm 35 and so healthy I don't even have a doctor. Yet my wife says I should have a physical every year. Seems to me that would be a waste of money.
—S. L., Houston

"I hear this all the time from guys in their 30s," says Michael Ponder, M.D., a family physician in Franklin, Virginia. "People move around so much these days that it's common for someone not to have a family doctor, and many men don't bother to look for one until something is seriously wrong." This is a mistake: You're likely to receive much better care from a doctor who knows your health history than from someone you picked out of the yellow pages during your ambulance ride.

If you don't have a doctor, find one and schedule a physical. "With a new patient, it's important to establish a baseline, to find out what is normal for that individual," says Dr. Ponder. "Once I learn about his lifestyle and family history, I can make specific recommendations and let him know what to watch out for."

After that initial exam, though, you may not have to see your doc for quite a while. Dr. Ponder suggests that men in good health have a complete physical every 3 to 5 years before age 40, every 2 years while in their 40s, and annually after age 50.

Monitoring Your Vision

My new job requires me to stare at a computer screen for hours at a time, and my eyesight seems to be deteriorating. Is this possible? What can I do, aside from changing jobs?
—B. A., New York City

"I've heard this a million times, but there is no evidence that computer screens emit anything harmful to vision," says Richard Lewis, M.D., an ophthalmologist at the Cullen Eye Institute at Baylor College of Medicine in Houston. The problem, says Dr. Lewis, is age: Close vision naturally begins to deteriorate at about 40, and people would rather blame their monitors than their failing organs. If this sounds familiar, suck it up and see an eye doctor. The interns will think your bifocals are cute.

Although computers don't damage vision, too many hours in front of the screen can cause eyestrain. It isn't dangerous, but it's uncomfortable. To avoid eyestrain, rest your eyes every 15 minutes by looking at distant objects—the women's cross-country team running by your office window, for instance. Some other tips: Color monitors are less fatiguing than black-and-white, and newer, higher-resolution monitors are gentler than older models. Fluorescent lights cause less glare than incandescent, and if you have a window in your office, invest in a glare screen.

Looking Past the Pain

Every once in a while I get an itchy, painful bump on my inner eyelid. What causes this, and how can I prevent it?
—J. N., Lansing, Mich.

Eyelid bumps, called chalazia, appear when the gland along the rim of the eyelid becomes clogged with normal secretions, says Rajiv Anand, M.D., associate professor of ophthalmology at the University of Texas in Dallas. This causes a local inflammation. To unblock the gland, apply a cotton ball soaked with hot water and hold it in place for 5 minutes. The bump should disappear in a few days. If the skin is red and sore, or if your vision is affected, see your eye doctor. You may have an infection that can be cleared up with prescription antibiotic eyedrops or ointment.

The Kindest Cut

How can I prevent ingrown toenails?
—M. R., Columbia, Miss.

Most ingrown toenails are caused by cutting the nail improperly, says Arnold Ravick, D.P.M., spokesman for the American Podiatric Medical Association. "Toenails should be cut straight across, so that the edge of the nail is on top of, rather than underneath, the skin," he says. "If you round them out the way you do your fingernails, the edges of the nail will grow into the skin." Ingrown nails can be aggravated by shoe rub—a problem in sports that emphasize lateral motion, such as tennis and basketball. Dr. Ravick recommends wearing sport-specific shoes and socks. You can also cut down on friction by applying a little petroleum jelly around the edge of the nail and covering it with an adhesive bandage. If you still get ingrown toenails, see a podiatrist, who can cut out a tiny piece of the nail and cauterize the spot so that it doesn't regrow.

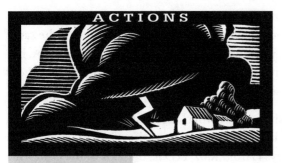

To live a long, healthy life, you need to be proactive. Simple things like visiting your doctor each year for a check-up, taking vitamins, and examining yourself for any suspicious lumps or moles could add years to your life. But there are also numerous things you can do to improve the *quality* of your life day-to-day. For example, eating garlic can help you avoid getting a cold, including all those annoying symptoms that go with it. Doing a simple stretch each day can help keep you from being laid up with a sore back. And paying attention to how your work space is set up can reduce your chances of getting a neckache. Read on for easy things you can do to live longer and, more important, live better.

1. **Increase your life expectancy with vitamin C.** Research from the UCLA School of Public Health indicates that men with high vitamin C intakes live longer than men with low intakes. A 35-year-old man who takes in 300 milligrams or more of C a day has a life expectancy 5.5 years longer than a man whose daily intake is less than 50 milligrams. Vitamin C may not get all the credit—high intake is often a sign of healthy habits—but getting enough C from fruits, vegetables, and supplements is definitely a smart move.

2. **Keep your date with your doc.** The male tendency to avoid doctors may be one reason women live longer than us. But seeing your doctor regularly can be the key to preventing death from a variety of causes, including colon cancer. A recent study tabulated that getting screened for the disease can help you live 2 to 3 years longer. Your screening should include an annual fecal occult blood test starting at age 50 (earlier if you have a family history of colon cancer) and a flexible sigmoidoscopy and a digital rectal exam (DRE) every 5 years. (You're probably already getting a yearly DRE for prostate cancer.)

3. **Get your blood flowing with a leg massage.** Sitting for a long time cuts off blood flow to your legs, so use massage to get that blood pumping again. While you're seated, cross your legs so that your right ankle rests on your left knee. Put one hand around your ankle, the other just above your knee. Move the hand that's around the ankle toward the knee with a gliding motion while applying slight pressure, and move the hand that's above the knee with the same motion toward the ankle so that your two hands meet halfway, says Robert A. Edwards, a licensed massage therapist and former director of the Somerset School of Massage Therapy in New Jersey. Then switch legs and repeat.

4. **Lay off the mouthwash if you're worried about bad breath.** Standard mouthwashes contain a lot of alcohol, which dries up the saliva in your mouth and makes your breath worse, says Harold Katz, D.D.S., director of the California Breath Clinic, which is based in Los Angeles. "Saliva is rich in oxygen, which keeps your mouth healthy and fresh," he explains. "Anaerobic bacteria thrive in a dry, low-oxygen environment and produce more sulfur compounds. Commercial mouthwashes dry your mouth and definitely don't help your breath. In fact, they make it worse." Instead, if you want to freshen your breath, rinse your mouth out with water, he advises.

5. **Take a snapshot of your arteries.** If your doctor has warned you about your cholesterol but you can't seem to lay off the three-cheese omelettes, post a picture of your arteries on the fridge. Cardiologist Jacques Barth, M.D., Ph.D., showed 210 patients ultrasound images of their blocked carotid arteries. The 105 who took copies home (including wallet-size snapshots) lost an average of 7 more pounds after 6 months, and their arterial blockages shrunk twice as much. "People are more likely to change when they can see exactly what cholesterol does," says Dr. Barth. Ask your doctor if you could benefit from this $150 to $200 ultrasound test.

6. **Eat chocolate for your health.** In what may be some of the best news science has given us in a long time, Harvard researchers who studied 7,841 male alumni found that those who ate candy bars regularly lived 1 year longer than guys who never touched the stuff. Don't use this as an excuse to begin a diet of Snickers and Tootsie Rolls, though. They also found that men who ate three or more sweets a week had a 30 percent higher risk of early death than men with more moderate habits—one to three candy bars per month. One theory in support of chocolate as health food: It contains phenols, antioxidants that help prevent fats in the blood from clogging arteries.

7. **When buying multivitamins, think generic.** "There's no reason to spend more than $4 to $5 a month on a multi," says Bonnie Liebman of the Center for Science in the Public Interest. "Generally, supplements sold at health food stores cost more than brand names, while generic supplements from large supermarkets or drugstore chains are the cheapest." There is often little difference between the effectiveness of a brand name and a generic supplement. In fact, they're often made by the same companies. Only the labels change.

8. **Get by with a little help from your friends.** Research now shows that hanging out with your pals can actually help you live longer. In fact, one study estimates that being social can gain you nearly a decade. People with very poor social connections live 4.5 years less than expected, while those with very good connections live 4.5 years longer.

9. **Inspect your neck when you shave.** Lumps on your neck can indicate either a simple infection or something more serious. Since men often see lumps before feeling them, inspect your neck when you're shaving; simply turn to the side and look for any unexplained bulges. If any lump is ¾ inch or more in diameter or lasts more than 2 weeks, see a doctor.

10. **Bend over backward for a strong back.** You can help to prevent back problems by doing a simple stretch. Stretching your back muscles helps you create a greater range of movement and also enhances the elasticity of your muscles and spinal joints, says Michael Reed Gach, Ph.D., founder of the Acupressure Institute in Berkeley, California, and author of *The Bum Back Book*. Here's a basic stretch and a good starting point: Stand with your hands behind your lower back for support and your knees slightly bent. Slowly bend backward, far enough to get a gentle stretch. Exhale as you bend. Then, come back up very slowly, keeping your knees bent, while you inhale. Do this exercise daily, stretching the spine several times. If this gentle exercise aggravates your back pain, stop it and consult a doctor or physical therapist, advises Dr. Gach.

11. **Raise a glass of OJ for heart health.** According to researchers at the University of Western Ontario, drinking orange juice can raise your "good" HDL cholesterol levels more than some medications. After 25 subjects drank three glasses of orange juice a day for 4 weeks, their HDL cholesterol levels rose by 21 percent. According to the study author, Elzbieta Kurowska, Ph.D., HDL cholesterol lowers your heart-disease risk by clearing harmful LDL cholesterol deposits from blood vessels. Both fresh squeezed OJ and from-concentrate varieties contain the phytochemicals that could be responsible for the results, says Dr. Kurowska.

12. **Scrape away bacteria.** Your tongue holds more bacteria than the floor of the men's room at Grand Central Station. "If you don't scrape your tongue after you brush your teeth, bacteria will instantly reinfest your mouth," says Perry R. Klokkevold, D.D.S., adjunct associate professor and clinical director at UCLA School of Dentistry. Buy a tongue scraper at the drugstore and take a few good swipes every morning and night. "Brushing your tongue isn't nearly as effective," he says.

13. Fight tartar without toothpaste. Brush your teeth with a dry tooth-brush once a day, advises Steven T. Bunn, D.D.S., a dentist in Alexandria, Virginia. Research has shown that people who dry-brush have significantly less tartar buildup than people who brush with toothpaste. Use gentle side-to-side strokes in which the brush is half on the gums and half on the tooth.

14. Don't let your office be a pain in the neck. A poorly arranged work-station is a common cause of neck and shoulder pain. You'll know that your key-board is at the proper height if your forearms are perfectly horizontal when your fingers rest on the keys. In addition, make sure your computer monitor is at the proper height to avoid muscle strain. "Be sure that your monitor is set at eye level. For proper positioning, the top of the monitor screen should be at or just below eye level," says Douglas Einstadter, M.D., assistant professor of medicine at Case Western Reserve University in Cleveland. If it is, your head will automatically be in a comfortable position.

15. Grab garlic to prevent colds. Garlic is one of nature's great immu-nizers, so it's a great defense strategy against the common cold. Crush or mash a fresh clove or two into anything from pesto to salad dressing, or just eat half a clove three times a day. A more sociable option when you actually get a cold is to take garlic capsules. A typical dosage is 300 milligrams, three times a day, for as long as cold symptoms last, says Adriane Fugh-Berman, M.D., former head of field investigations for the Office of Alternative Medicine at the National Insti-tutes of Health and author of *Alternative Medicine: What Works.*

6

MENTAL
TOUGHNESS

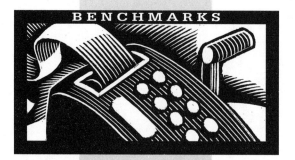

■ Average time in minutes it takes for executives to decide whether a candidate is right for a job: 16

■ Percentage of instances where the last interviewee gets the job: 56

■ Percentage of men who claim to be happiest when they're alone: 66

■ Percentage of men 18 to 49 years old who say it's harder to be a man now than it was 20 years ago: 60

■ Ranking of the following rule: Don't Panic: 1

■ Best time of day to testify in court: 9:00 to 10:00 A.M.

■ Chances that listening to Mozart will make you smarter: 0

■ Ratio by which parents report perceived stress of watching their kids compete compared to undergoing surgery themselves: 1:1

■ Percentage of people who believe "being there through thick and thin" is an admirable quality: 89

■ Percentage of people who believe "being willing to do the right thing" is an admirable quality: 83

■ Percentage of people who believe "putting family ahead of work" is an admirable quality: 82

■ Percentage of people who believe "the ability to keep a secret" is an admirable quality: 72

■ Rank of self-confidence as a factor for happiness in the United States: 1

■ Percentage chance your parents will live longer if you maintain very close personal ties with them: 40

■ Percentage of Americans suffering from social phobias: 13

■ Number of hours of lost leisure time per week since the 1970s: 6.8

■ Percentage by which people with moderate anger are likely to have an acute/fatal heart attack as compared with those with cooler tempers: 35

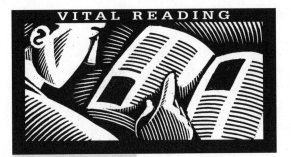

Your Body's Stress S.O.S.

Watch out for these signs that stress may be getting the better of you.

Problems are best solved by avoiding them in the first place. Leave the bar before a fight, apologize before she cries, sneak out before they pass the collection plate. But there's one problem we can't avoid, simply because we can't see it. It's invisible. It's stress. It may be all around us, but where exactly is it?

It's true that stress makes itself known in a number of explicit ways. But when we notice it, it's often too late to do anything. By then we've already snapped at our boss or yelled at our girlfriend. Or both, depending on their state of undress when we walked in on them.

You can avoid all that if you detect stress before it grows real claws. By spotting these hidden signs of growing anxiety, you can cut the tension before it cuts you.

Your biceps are sore, even though you haven't worked out in 2 weeks. When you're stressed, certain hormones, such as adrenaline (epinephrine), tighten all your muscles, not just your neck and shoulders, which are the ones we normally associate with stress. "When your muscles remain tense for extended periods of time, you feel soreness," says Allen Elkin, Ph.D., director of the Stress Management and Counseling Center in New York City.

What to do about it: Flex. Tighten and contract your muscles, starting with your calves and moving up to your shoulders and neck. The contracting and relaxing should help relieve soreness, says Steven Edwards, Ph.D., professor of health psychology at Oklahoma State University in Stillwater. If you're in a jam at work, try squeezing your thumb and index finger together. This move won't solve any problems, but it may ease your tension enough to let you see in a much better light what has you so stressed.

You sleep 8 hours a night, but still feel tired. Getting enough sleep doesn't mean you're getting enough rest. Stress keeps your mind wide awake and unable to relax, even while you're sleeping. That's because it keeps you from attaining your most restful state during sleep, which can leave you feeling groggy even after a full night in bed.

What to do about it: Get hot. "A shower or hot bath before bed will raise your body's temperature. Your temperature will then fall faster when you crawl into bed, so you'll have a deeper sleep," says Ed Stepanski, Ph.D., a sleep expert at Rush-Presbyterian St. Luke's medical center in Chicago. Soak 30 minutes for maximum effectiveness, and don't eat anything afterward. Your body won't rest for the first half of the night if it's trying to digest food.

You've lost your desire to masturbate. A loss of libido—especially quickie, on-your-own-time libido—could be a psychological reaction to stress. "When you're subconsciously worried about other things, you don't have the desire to seek out pleasure in any form," Dr. Elkin notes. Oddly, it's when you're stressed out that sex is needed most—it's one of the body's best methods of releasing endorphins and reducing tension.

What to do about it: Give your body what it needs, even if it takes a little effort. "Creating a fantasy in your mind when it's not possible to act on it builds up stimulation throughout the day," says Joel Block, Ph.D., a psychologist and the author of *Secrets of Better Sex.* In other words, think about sex at work. That builds up sexual tension, so when you arrive home, the urge will be strong enough to overpower any stress that was initially blocking its path. Then find your partner—or a Spanish soap opera.

You bounced two checks last month. Stress can affect your concentration, and it can also make you clumsy, lazy, and all-around cement-headed. Stress often manifests itself in mathematical mistakes or transposition of numbers, says Herbert Benson, M.D., professor of behavioral medicine at Harvard Medical School. If you're making more mistakes than usual, don't worry. You're not getting dumber, you're probably not developing Alzheimer's, and it's not the beer, either. It's your brain telling you to slow down.

What to do about it: As soon as you receive a work assignment, make a schedule. "One of the biggest reasons people make mistakes at work is that they procrastinate, then work too quickly," says Kenneth De Meuse, Ph.D., professor of management at the University of Wisconsin in Madison. You learned this hazardous practice in college (it was called "cramming"), and back then it worked out fine. But that was when you were 18, when staying up all night eating pizza and reading Balzac was kind of fun. You're a grown-up now. Buy a day planner.

You go through a pack of gum every morning. Fingernail-biting and foot-tapping may be the telltale habits of anxious men, but any kind of repetitive motion—chewing gum, biting your pen, picking your nose—is your body's sub-conscious way of trying to relax.

What to do about it: Your body wants repetition? Give it repetition. Go to a driving range, shoot 100 free throws, or climb some stairs. Activities that involve repetition relieve tension better than those that require more varied activities—a round of golf or a game of one-on-one. "The repetition relaxes your body, stops the production of stress-causing hormones, and returns your body to normal," explains Dr. Benson.

You ignore your hobbies. When you're stressed, it's completely normal and sensible to spend most of your time focused on what's causing the stress. But what if that's at the expense of activities that might actually help you relax? "Handling all the perceived negatives in your life leaves little room for interacting with people or enjoying outside activities," points out Louise Holt, Ph.D., a California psychologist.

What to do about it: Free up time by doing jobs once and only once. The biggest waste of time in people's lives is retracing steps, says Carol Goldberg, Ph.D., a stress management specialist. If you have to go to the barber, pick up dry cleaning, and hit the store, do it all in one trip. This keeps you from re-peating routes and wasting time. At work, do the same. Break projects down to their simplest components and move from one step to the next, or you'll simply repeat the steps you've already completed. This leaves room to return to your favorite hobby, whether it's playing poker, shooting pool, or robbing conve-nience stores.

You watch TV more and read less. Television requires little of what reading demands: concentration. Stress hinders your ability to focus, so it's no wonder you're watching other people do things instead of doing something yourself. Staring passively at images is much more soothing than processing words, and when your mind is taxed, it needs to relax. So you'll watch anything, even cooking shows.

What to do about it: We're not going to knock television. TV, in our opinion, is one of the greatest stress-reducers known to man, second only to skeet shooting. But at some point you have to ask yourself whether you're watching TV to relax or to escape some nagging anxiety. If it's the latter, forcing yourself to read your usual novels instead of staring at the tube won't do you any good, says Daniel Alkon, M.D., of the National Institutes of Health. "You'll only have a harder time concentrating because you'll be distracted," he says. You need to re-build your concentration levels. Instead of tackling Tolstoy, start with something simplistic, like newspaper articles or pro athletes' autobiographies.

Depression in the Big Leagues

Major League pitcher Pete Harnisch's battle with depression proves that none of us are immune to mental illness.

After shoulder surgery and back-to-back losing seasons, Pete Harnisch, a pitcher for the New York Mets, looked at 1997 as a make-or-break year. He broke.

It wasn't a spectacular injury that sidelined him. It was clinical depression, a disease that affects about 6.3 million men every year. Depression is serious—even deadly—if untreated; and it's often untreated. Many men are reluctant to seek the help they need, believing depression strikes only simpering neurotics and angry loners. A bull of a man, known among his teammates as a jokester, Harnisch had everything a guy could want—money, fame, a beautiful wife, a dream job. But a sweet lifestyle can't inoculate you against depression any more than it can prevent the flu. "If you're walking down the street thinking it can't happen to you, you're kidding yourself," Harnisch says. "I never thought it would happen to me."

Harnisch's depression began in spring training, with mild but persistent insomnia, lightheadedness, cold sweats, and anxiety. Since he'd recently quit chewing tobacco, he assumed his symptoms were the result of nicotine withdrawal. He did what most guys do—ignored the problems, figuring they'd go away. But they got worse daily. "I lost my personality," he says. "I didn't feel like talking to anyone. I didn't feel like golfing, which normally I love. I lost my appetite—I didn't even want pizza." Yes, pizza. What Harnisch didn't know was that he had an imbalance of mood-regulating chemicals in his brain. An imbalance can cause the kind of symptoms Harnisch was experiencing, as well as severe mood swings, thoughts of death and suicide, loss of enthusiasm for usual activities, panic attacks, phobias, and mind-numbing lows.

He fought through the symptoms until April's season opener in San Diego. "Then it got to the point where I was having trouble functioning, and I wasn't sure I could do my job," he says.

He confided in Bobby Valentine, the Mets manager, telling him he felt shaky and unsure of himself. Valentine accused him of being a coward, says Harnisch, reinforcing the cliché: Something bothering you? Rub it with a brick.

But you can no more "get over" clinical depression than you can a brain tumor.

Harnisch could have felt shame—being called a coward by your coach is verbal castration—but instead he decided to see a doctor. After gutting out five innings in the Mets' season-opening loss to San Diego, Harnisch flew east.

It took doctors in New York only a day to diagnose his depression. Whether it was triggered by the stress of another season, nicotine withdrawal, heredity (his family has a history of the disease), a virus, or some other cause isn't known. But it was real.

"I felt so bad, I wasn't worried about what people would think. I was worried about what was happening to me," Harnisch says. "It was a relief to know the source, put a name to it, and find out there was stuff I could do to get better."

Away from the Game

For the first time in 25 years, Harnisch spent a summer without baseball, pouring his energy into recovery. Step one: finding the right antidepressant medication. Though drugs are effective for 80 to 90 percent of depression sufferers, determining which one will work isn't easy. You can pick from five selective serotonin reuptake inhibitors (SSRIs)—the best medicines to fight the disease—but there's no way to tell which, if any, will produce results. Complicating matters: Antidepressants take 3 to 4 weeks to work. Patients can spend months searching for the proper drug and dosage.

Harnisch's case was typical. He tried another SSRI before having success with Paxil. After he'd been on the medication for 3 weeks, his anxiety lessened, his mood picked up—he even liked pizza again. Just as important, he experienced none of the side effects (including sexual dysfunction and insomnia) commonly caused by SSRIs. Harnisch also began talk therapy with a psychiatrist. He wasn't looking to blame his parents or anyone else for his crash, and he was savvy enough to know that "any doctor who tries to make you someone you're not is irresponsible." Instead, he looked for ways to handle his symptoms and to better understand his own psyche, especially his reactions to the ups and downs of his pressure-filled career.

When it comes to baseball, Harnisch now focuses on the one element he can control—preparation. "To some degree, I don't give a crap anymore about the outcome of a baseball game," he says. "But in an odd way I care more because I put everything I have into getting ready to pitch. I'm just as determined to win, but I don't get as pissed off over one run or one loss."

And he no longer lets the game affect how he treats his friends or his wife, Donna. "She's the one who got me out of bed and moving when I felt awful," Harnisch says. "You'd really be crazy to try and take on depression by yourself."

Returning to the Mound

The next step for Harnisch was to rebuild himself physically—he lost 40 pounds during the ordeal. Still, he had to ease his way back into shape. Though exercise is often touted as a "cure" for low-level depression, it can make certain symptoms, such as fatigue and anxiety, worse if it's overdone. "At first I couldn't do more than 10 minutes on the stair-climbing machine, and I was used to doing an hour," he says. "But slowly my strength and energy came back."

By August of 1997, Harnisch felt good enough for a late-season return to the Mets. But throwing a baseball turned out to be the easiest part. "I felt like my teammates were watching me more closely, but really it was me feeling awkward, not them," he says. "I like to tease guys, but I just didn't feel as comfortable doing it when I first came back. After a little while, though, we started screwing around and joking like we used to."

Things didn't go as smoothly with Valentine, and it became apparent that the two wouldn't be able to mend their relationship. Harnisch was traded to Milwaukee in September, and he started four games for the Brewers, finishing with a 1-0 record. He's had even greater success pitching for Cincinnati. "It was a relief to get back on the mound. I felt like myself again," he says.

"If It Comes Back, I'll Deal with It"

Some patients stay on antidepressants to regulate their moods, but Harnisch was among those able to give up their medications once their brain chemistries return to normal. After 7 months of Paxil and therapy, doctors weaned him from both.

Though fully recovered, Harnisch says there's one lasting legacy of his depression: a wormhole of doubt where before none existed. "Pitching in big games, taking on situations that make you nervous, that's a challenge when you've been through depression, because a small part of you always wonders how you'll react," he says.

For now, Harnisch feels as if he's beaten clinical depression, but he knows that recurrence is common—about 50 percent—and that someday he may have to face the disease again. "If it comes back, it comes back," he says. "I'll deal with it."

Outsmart Job Stress

No matter what type of job you have, there's a stress-busting activity that will help you clear your mind.

Stress is like a tight muscle: You have to stretch it in the opposite direction to relieve the tension. So relax by using the skills you ignore in your job. This will pull you out of the rut you've dug for yourself, and it will call on parts of your brain that, frankly, could use a little exercise. The benefit: When you kick back, you'll bounce back, and you'll have fewer empties to bring to the recycling center.

Your stress: You make big decisions

Your outlet: Take an art or music class

As the boss who decides the fate of the company or the surgeon who decides the fate of the person lying on the table, you're constantly doing the heavy cerebral lifting. The counterbalance to those neurons firing to handle analytical work is something that taxes the artistic region of your brain. "Music is a good stress release for someone whose decisions are constantly under scrutiny, because there's no objective means of evaluation," says James Campbell Quick, Ph.D., a psychologist at the University of Texas at Arlington. As long as you're practicing alone, of course.

Your stress: You work with deadlines

Your outlet: Aimless wandering

In deadline situations, your body releases adrenaline—a chemical messenger that sharpens your senses so you can finish the job. But that one-dimensional project probably means that you're neglecting other important things in your life, like your family or your health. And that frustration can make you one pissed-off professional.

"Backpacking is the perfect antidote because it's slow and methodical," says Dr. Quick. Unlike running, which is measured in time, or even fishing, which has surges of excitement during the strike and catch, backpacking forces you to slow down. As long as you're not trying to bag a peak or outsmart a hungry bear, hiking rests the part of your brain that triggers the adrenaline response. By looking at the trees and the trail, you learn to focus on many elements, not just one.

Your stress: You spend your week being nice to people

Your outlet: Hitting people—hard

As a salesman, a waiter, or a PR guy, you spend most of your time giving the outward appearance of being charming, positive, and happy. The effect? You grow frustrated with people who don't buy what you're selling or agitated with diners who leave lousy tips. If you don't relieve your pent-up emotions—and let's face it, the busboy doesn't want to hear your troubles—they'll be stored in your body as muscle tension. Your outlet should let you be as agitated as you damn well please. "When you're boxing, the flip side of being in control can come out," Dr. Quick says. Hitting a punching bag (whether it's leather or human) gives you a kinetic release that burns up the fuel of the stress response—glucose—that you've accumulated all week.

Your stress: Repetitive work

Your outlet: Become a beer, wine, or food snob

If your job is one-dimensional, you're probably clogging up the part of your brain that functions all day, whether it's the one that writes reports, tightens bolts, or crunches numbers. By picking an activity that works all of your senses—wine tasting, beer brewing, or competing in a barbecue cookoff—you give that part of your brain a chance to wind down while you stimulate other parts. "Something that engages your senses allows you to get out of your head and focus on smell, taste, touch, sight," says Lou Perrott, Ph.D., a business psychologist. Any activity that stimulates smell and taste helps divert the attention you normally spend on your one-track job.

Your stress: The job you have, as pleasant as it is, doesn't allow upward mobility

Your outlet: Compete on the playing field

Maybe you're a teacher who doesn't want to become a principal. Or maybe you're a small-business owner who has no position to rise into. Whatever the case, you're not moving toward a well-defined goal. If that makes you feel complacent and unchallenged, it can be frustrating to watch friends and family move up in the corporate world. As an antidote, you need an outlet that offers intense competition. Individual sports, such as cycling and running, are better than team sports because you're in full control of how well and how fast you progress. "Marathons are good because you can't train for one in a week. You control how long and hard you train," says Dr. Perrott. The tactics of running a race not only provide an outlet for your competitive side, they also teach you when to conserve energy, when to make a move, and when to hang behind the pack.

Your stress: You spend most of your workday with strangers

Your outlet: Join the club

If you're surrounded by people you have nothing in common with (maybe you're the computer guy at a hospital), you need to relax with people you can relate to. By taking a continuing education class in something you care about, you'll be spending time with people who share your interests. "What you're looking for as an antidote to difficult relationships are therapeutic, healthy, and easy relationships," Dr. Quick says. As long as you don't take the class for a grade, that should do the trick.

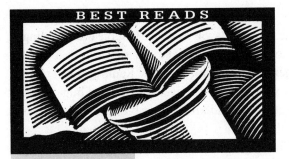

Sound Smarter Than You Are

Quantum physics. The economic history of the Pacific island of Vanuatu. The latest Clive Cussler book. Have you ever found yourself in a conversation where the topic changed to something you knew nothing about? Of course you have. Now you could try and fake an opinion and hope that nobody calls you on your obvious ignorance. You could also simply admit that you're out of your league. Or, better yet, you can take the advice found in the following excerpt from Guy Knowledge *(Rodale). Authors Larry Keller, Christian Millman, and the editors of* Men's Health *Books offer solid strategies on how to impress others even when you don't have a clue what they're talking about.*

Eddie the plumber used to drink beer with Raymond D. Strother, a partner in Strother, Duffy, Strother, a political consulting firm in Washington, D.C. At various times in his career, Strother has given political advice to Bill Clinton, Al Gore, Gary Hart, and many, many others. He's also the vice president of the American Association of Political Consultants.

Strother recounts, "One day, Eddie said to me, 'Look, I'm not very smart, and I don't know many words. Is there anything you can recommend to me so I don't seem as dumb as I feel?' I said, 'Well, Eddie, that's easy. Do what intellectuals do.'"

So, what do intellectuals do?

"I said, 'Eddie, just tell them it's relative,'" says Strother. If you're asked for an opinion, on any topic, the answer is the same. It's relative. Eddie tried that and was awestruck.

Eddie was so awestruck, in fact, that he came back to Strother for additional advice. He really wanted to impress his boss. Strother taught him a word—viscosity. Eddie, being a plumber, was able to use a word like viscosity to describe thick things going down a drain.

"He went around trying to find ways to work the word *viscosity* into things," recalls Strother. It impressed the hell out of Eddie's boss.

The moral of this story: Sounding smarter than you are is probably much easier than you think.

All of the People, Some of the Time

Maybe you don't qualify for Mensa. Maybe you have trouble even spelling it. No matter. Here are some tips to raise your perceived IQ.

Bone up. Ray Suarez, former host of National Public Radio's *Talk of the Nation*, was faced with a two-hour show, four days a week, covering a huge number of topics. Still, he always managed to sound knowledgeable, even when it was a topic that was way out of his field. How?

Homework. "The method for prep is to not try to learn everything the night before," he explains. "That would be like trying to cram for a final in a class you've never attended."

He knew what topics were likely to come up and started scanning the papers and television for information. You can do the same. If you know you have a dinner party with the boss and his florist friends, check out some books on flower arranging. If you're going to a big bluegrass revival concert, borrow a few compact discs from the library and read the dust jackets. Again, the idea is to know a few things about the topic well enough to carry on an intelligent conversation about them.

Find an expert. When something really big happens in the world, what do the talking heads on TV do? They ask experts to tell us what it all means. You can do the same. If a big event is coming up and you know nothing about it, find someone who does, says William L. Benoit, Ph.D., professor of communication at the University of Missouri in Columbia.

"You can't know everything about everything," he says. Find someone who knows the score and ask him to give you a nutshell description of the important issues at hand. Odds are, he'll be flattered that you thought highly enough of him to ask his opinion.

Take your time. When someone throws you a conversational curveball, don't blurt out the first thing that pops into your head. There's no time limit on answers. And there are two hidden benefits in going slow. "One, you might think of something to say," says Dr. Benoit. "Two, people may get the impression that you're being thoughtful." Little do they know that you're trying to figure out how to scratch unobtrusively.

Hold your ground. As the host of the popular game show *Jeopardy!*, Alex Trebek makes a living appearing smart. True, he really *is* smart, but even he estimates that he knows only about two-thirds of the material on the show. So what happens when conversations in his real life wander into the few areas where he isn't knowledgeable? One trick Trebek uses is to substitute clever humor in place of actual knowledge and steer the talk back to familiar ground.

For example, if the discussion turns to the philosophical meaning of sanity, Trebek suggests saying: "I love the sanatee. I go to see them in the Florida waters all the time."

Here's another variation on the same theme. Say the bleeding heart historians start talking about Dame Edith Cavell, the noted English nurse executed by Germans in World War I. You could casually say, "Enos Cabell? I think the Dodgers lost a great third baseman when he retired." Not only do you save face, you get to turn the talk to baseball.

"I can do stuff like this hoping that the stupid thing that I'm saying will be recognized as such by intelligent people because they know that I know better," says Trebek. Plus, unlike on *Jeopardy!*, you get extra points for creativity.

Recognize that sometimes, the most intelligent thing you can say is nothing at all. Learn to manage your silences; doing so can be much better than speaking, says Strother.

It's a sentiment echoed by Dr. Benoit. If you're in an unfamiliar situation, he says, mum is your most useful word. "If you're talking a lot and grasping at straws, you'll say things that are contradictory," he says. "Clearly, that doesn't make you look smarter."

Replace your words with knowing nods, bemused smiles, and thoughtful glances.

But Not All of the People All of the Time

Strother once worked on the campaign of a candidate for governor of Louisiana. "This guy was so dumb that he once bragged to me how he went all the way through law school and never once in his life finished a whole book," says Strother.

He taught his gubernatorial candidate all the tricks. The candidate even used the word "viscosity" in his television ads. He was always photographed and filmed in the company of Louisiana's brightest minds: scientists, civic leaders, top businessmen. And for months, he was leading in the polls. Then, as election day neared, the politico began to drop. He ran second, then third, finally ending up last. Curious and frustrated, Strother conducted some exit polls.

"The reason my guy slipped to fourth was because people didn't think he was smart enough," recalls Strother. There's a valuable lesson here. Louisiana political campaigns run for about a year and a half. By the time voting day rolled around, people had the man figured out.

There's a statute of limitations on your smart act. Eventually, people will see through it. If you're faking intelligence, consider yourself on a dive-bombing mission. Fly in there, hit 'em with all your armament, and then get the heck out of there before they catch on.

Oh, and don't run for governor.

The Respect of Your Peers

Sometimes working in an office can seem like you're playing in the NHL. While a rookie is getting checked against the boards, your coworkers are questioning your paycheck in the boardroom. Just got a great promotion and a cushy corner office? Learn what's behind the jealous looks of your former cubicle-mates. Noticed that your peers' respect for you seems to be dwindling? Identify some key phrases in your speech that could be robbing you of your authority. In this excerpt from Command Respect *(Rodale), Perry Garfinkel, Brian Paul Kaufman, and the editors of* Men's Health *Books offer advice to help you survive—and thrive among—your coworkers.*

It was the novelist and critic Gore Vidal who once commented: "Whenever a friend succeeds, a little something in me dies." Admit it, you know the feeling. We all do. And perhaps nowhere is that more true than in the workplace.

As any newly minted vice-president will tell you, hard work and great ideas will help land you not only an executive parking spot but also the scornful looks of some jealous peers. It seems unfair that the very conduct that earns you the respect of your boss and a fast-track to promotion also can result in backbiting and jealousy among your coworkers. But then, nobody ever said life is fair.

Jealousy may be the main factor that can rob you of the respect of your coworkers, but it certainly isn't the only one. Constant complaining, talking about people behind their backs, and contrasting personal styles also can breed disrespect. There are, however, actions you can take today to counter these common workplace maladies so that you are judged worthy of respect by the jury of your peers.

Promoting Harmony

All of your hard work finally paid off. You've been promoted. And suddenly, the guys you play hoops with at lunchtime each week treat you differently. What you sense isn't respect. It's more like . . . resentment. What's going on? After all, if one of them had gotten the promotion, you'd be happy for them. Wouldn't you?

Even among friends, the success of one can fuel insecurity in another. "All jealous people basically feel they're not as good as others," says Paul Hauck, Ph.D., a psychologist in Rock Island, Illinois, and author of *Overcoming the Rating Game*.

Some of your peers see your achievement and feel like there must be something lacking in themselves. "They rate themselves by your success," Dr. Hauck says. "'He got the promotion, I didn't. He is better than I am. I am insanely jealous of that other person. Why didn't it happen to me?' They believe that getting a promotion makes you a better person."

One of the ways you can show that you're worthy of your new title is by handling the situation with skill. Here are a few suggestions.

Lose the cape. As tempting as it may be to display your superhuman skills and ambitions to these lesser mortals, it's the last thing you want to do. "You need to exude the idea that you're no better than they," Dr. Hauck says. "Underplay your success if you can."

Encourage the envious. Say you have a buddy who's happy for you, but disappointed in his own apparent lack of success. He will respect you even more if you take the time to encourage him. Dr. Hauck suggests telling him, "I like the stuff you're doing. If it were up to me, you'd be next."

Corner the market on motivation. Behind almost every great fighter is a great cornerman, a trainer who prepares his boxer for success and keeps him motivated and focused during the bout. Even if you're now in the corner office, you can knock out office jealousy by making it clear to a disgruntled coworker that you're in his corner. "Your attitude and actions should underscore the idea that you'd like to help move him ahead in his career as much as you can," says Dr. Hauck.

Corral Complaining

If you're the kind of guy who confuses honesty with bitching and moaning, break out your violin: People not only don't respect you but they don't like you, and they can see you coming a mile away. "These are the attributes that people associate with complainers: negativity, moodiness, dogmatism, and—surprise—pessimism," says Robin Kowalski, Ph.D., associate professor of psychology at Western Carolina University in Cullowhee, North Carolina. "And if you exhibit those kinds of characteristics, according to our research, you're going to be pretty well disliked."

So why do some guys complain? It turns out that the old *Saturday Night Live* sketch about an annoying family known as The Whiners was probably right on the money. Complaining is probably, in part, another charming parental legacy. "If your parents were chronic complainers, then in all likelihood you're going to have some of those traits," Dr. Kowalski says.

But you can break the habit. Here are three steps Dr. Kowalski recommends.

Find someone who cares. If you must complain, for Pete's sake, find someone who cares and isn't going to blab the sad tale all over creation. "I think the best advice is to be more discriminating," Dr. Kowalski says. "You don't want to alienate everyone you talk to. If you're discriminating, not only do you have to think about whom you're going to complain to but you also might even reconsider complaining entirely."

Get a real greeting. If your peers dart into their offices and cubicles as you walk past, it might be because you've failed to master Greeting 101. For example, if Walter from marketing says, "How are you?" he doesn't really want to hear about your ingrown toenails or the fact that the transmission fell out of your minivan on your way to Disney World. In fact, there's a good chance that the only reason Walter asked you how you are was to give *himself* an opportunity to brag about his trip to Barbados with his new girlfriend, who—by the way—was just named Ms. September. Now that you know the game, simply answer "Great" and keep moving. If you're greeting others, "Good to see you" is a lot less nosy than "How are you?" and gives people a warm fuzzy—plus, *you'll* get fewer sob stories.

Get a clue. Suppose you unload your misery on the guy in the next dump truck—a tale of woe so dreadful that even this tattoo-wearing, beer-drinking behemoth is speechless. When the big guy finally weighs in with his opinion, it's a good idea just to listen carefully and then shut up. "A woman will stand there and keep listening, but the man will give you a problem-solving response and expect you to deal with it," Dr. Kowalski says. "If you keep complaining, it's like . . . 'I already told you what to do, man. Move on.'"

Making It Work

There are other things you can do to enhance the respect of your peers. There also are things you can *not* do that will boost your standing. It's important to know the difference. Here are four suggestions from our experts.

Keep your ears open. You don't have to become the office psychologist or spend countless hours listening to sob stories. But guys who are willing to listen to their peers are so rare, you'll earn respect practically by default.

"Most people are poor listeners," says organizational psychologist Dr. Darrel W. Ray. "There is a tremendous amount of miscommunication that takes place in American business. People just don't want to listen to each other. And that leads to rudeness and disrespect . . . the whole social system breaks down."

Abolish "aboutism." What's worse than pretending someone doesn't exist? How about talking about them behind their back, a practice Dr. Ray calls aboutism.

"It's rampant in most workplaces. We all do it in the lunchroom and the break room, and we do it after work . . . during meetings and after meetings," he says. "Talking about people, complaining about them, rather than going to that person. In order to gain respect, you cannot engage in that kind of behavior. It destroys respect of any kind."

Be a behavioral scientist. You—and your stomach—would probably be pretty upset if your coworker showed up an hour late to relieve you for your dinner break. But you'll have a better chance of helping him change if you can focus on his behavior rather than on him. "If I say, 'You didn't get back until 8:10 P.M.,' that is behavioral. You can observe that. But if I say, 'Bob, you're always late coming back from break,' that is not behavioral. Focus on what the behavior was and not the person. It's not the person that's bad. It's the behavior that hurts the company or hurts the team," says Dr. Ray.

Respect the other guy's style. Put two extremely talented, yet very different, people together and two things can happen. They can complement and challenge each other, producing work that exceeds what either could do individually (see Lennon and McCartney), or they could wind up at each other's throats, unable to stand even being in the same room together (see Lennon and McCartney). The key is to respect each other's differences and styles.

"You have to be somewhat understanding of the other's quirks and habits, moods, their best times to work, things like that," says Robert R. Butterworth, Ph.D., a trauma consultant and president of International Trauma Associates in Los Angeles.

If side-by-side collaboration is too intense, maybe that's why God invented fax machines and modems.

Belittlers, Be Gone

One common way we let respect slip away is by using phrases that communications consultant George Walther calls belittlers.

"The idea of power talking isn't that you boost yourself and make yourself better than you are but, rather, that you give yourself appropriate credit," Walther says. "And you can't do that when you are belittling yourself." Two of the most common belittlers are:

- "I'm just . . ." You can really bring yourself down a few notches in the eyes of your peers by frequently saying, "I'm just (fill in the blank)." "There is no reason to ever say, 'I am just anything,'" Walther advises. "It's quite common for a secretary taking a message to say, 'Well, gee, I don't know his availability. I'm just his assistant.' Compare that to 'I'm his assistant. I will be glad to check his availability and get back to you.' There's no question which sounds better."
- "You'll have to excuse . . ." You can really raise questions about your competency by using this phrase. It does not one but two detrimental things: It draws attention to the things that you didn't want the other person to notice *and*, at no extra charge, makes it look like you feel guilty. "They may not have thought, 'My gosh, what a mess this is!' but they will when you say, 'Oh, you'll have to excuse the condition of my office.' I say fix it or forget about it. If you don't like the way your office looks, either clean it up or stop apologizing to others and just get on with your life. Odds are they aren't going to notice anyway," Walther says.

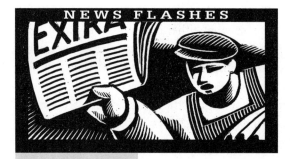

Benching Less Helps to Beat Stress

MADISON, Wis.—A University of Wisconsin study shows that moderate weight lifting elevates mood better than strenuous lifting. Researchers asked one group to lift weights for 30 minutes at 80 percent of their maximum. A second group pumped for 30 minutes at 50 percent, and a third watched an exercise video. Only the moderate exercisers improved their mood—they felt up to 50 percent less tension, depression, and anger. Additional research is needed to determine why lifting less weight is more effective.

Testosterone May Lead to Higher Rates of Depression

WASHINGTON, D.C.—A testosterone patch may help a flagging libido, but it won't do much for your mood. New research suggests that high levels of testosterone may make men depressed. In a study published in the *Journal of Health and Social Behavior*, researchers tested 4,393 men and found that those with higher levels of testosterone had up to three times the depression rate of men with normal levels. Alan Booth, Ph.D., the lead study author, suggests that men on supplemental testosterone keep an eye out for signs of depression, such as sudden weight loss and chronic lethargy.

It May Be Healthy to Chuckle at Others

LOMA LINDA, Calif.—You've heard for years that laughter is the best medicine. Now there's proof. Half of a group of 48 heart-attack survivors watched a comedy video of their choice for 30 minutes a day for a year. The other half weren't allowed to watch anything funny. After 12 months, only two patients in the first group had suffered another heart attack, compared with 10 in the second group. "Daily laughter seems to help restore the brain neurotransmitters that help you cope with stress," says study author Stanley Tan, M.D., Ph.D., of Loma Linda University.

Sleeping In Longer May Beat Stress

LONDON—There are about 6,000 good reasons to stay in bed, but here's one that doesn't involve sponge baths. Stress levels are lower in people who wake up later than 7:21 A.M., according to researchers at London's University of Westminster who measured the stress hormone cortisol in 42 people. "The surge in cortisol isn't influenced by whether a person wakes up by alarm. It's influenced by your body clock," says Angela Clow, Ph.D. *Note:* They didn't test stress levels of those fired for being late to work.

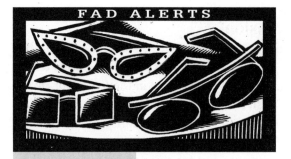

S-adenosyl-l-methionine (SAM-e)

 S-adenosyl-l-methionine (or SAM-e, for short) is a compound that your body produces from the amino acid methionine. It's a best-selling supplement that's being touted as a natural depression fighter more potent than St. John's wort. Thirty 200-milligram pills cost about $30.

One theory is that, like Prozac, SAM-e increases the levels of brain chemicals such as serotonin, says Maurizio Fava, M.D., a psychiatrist at Massachusetts General Hospital who has conducted three studies on the compound. In a review of 13 European published studies involving 200 people, 61 percent of those who took 1,600 milligrams of SAM-e daily had relief from depression, compared with 59 percent who took the prescription drug imipramine (Tofranil) and 22 percent taking a placebo. "These small studies only lasted up to 3 weeks, which is too short to judge the effectiveness of antidepressants," cautions Lorrin Koran, M.D., a psychiatrist at Stanford University.

Depression is a serious medical problem, so you should see a doctor. And if you need an antidepressant, don't expect him to recommend an over-the-counter pill. "SAM-e just isn't as proven as drugs like Prozac," says Dr. Fava. If prescription drugs fail to work, however, SAM-e is an option to discuss with your doctor.

Classical Music for Improved Cognition

Buy classical CDs if you enjoy them, but don't expect them to help you get into law school. Contrary to popular belief, listening to Mozart doesn't make you smarter. A few years ago, two studies showed that college students performed better on cognitive tests after listening to Mozart. But when Appalachian State University researchers in Boone, North Carolina, recently duplicated one of these studies, they found that 125 adults who listened to Mozart were no better at solving puzzles than a control group.

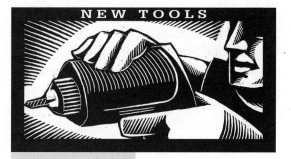

Less Damage from Strokes

Laser Treatment for Blood Clots

In less than 1 minute, a tiny experimental laser can destroy the blood clots that cause strokes. Conventional clot-busting drug treatments can take up to 2 hours. The new device could mean less brain damage and more lives saved, says lead researcher Wayne M. Clark, M.D., director of the Oregon Stroke Center in Portland.

The laser could one day be widely used to break up large clots in major arteries—clots that could otherwise cause quick, severe strokes. Clot-dissolving drugs may remain the treatment of choice for less-severe attacks in smaller blood vessels where the laser cannot reach, Dr. Clark notes. The laser is currently undergoing safety tests in humans, and it could be available within 5 years.

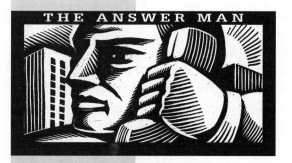

Punching Out the Clock

I stay up late on weekends. But even if I sleep for 8 hours afterward, I'm still tired. Why?
—L. C., Omaha, Neb.

Unlike your bedside clock, the dials of your internal timer can't just be spun to fit your partying schedule. "Even if you try to sleep the same number of hours, you won't feel as refreshed because your biological clock is out of sync with your irregular sleep habits," says James B. Maas, Ph.D., a psychology and sleep specialist at Cornell University in Ithaca, New York. "Biologically speaking, you're probably waking up smack in the middle of the early-afternoon low point in alertness." You're better off waking up at your normal hour and slinking off for a power nap later in the day.

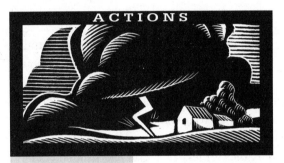

ACTIONS

It's easy to find workouts and health tips for your body. But what about that all-important driver at the helm—your mind? In today's world, being mentally sharp can make the difference between being the guy in the corner office and being the guy in the mail room. Hit the mental gym with the following tips and hints.

1. When you need some Zzzs, think valerian. A tired mind is a groggy mind. The best fix? A restful night in the sack. The herb valerian offers mild tranquilizing effects and has been shown to help people fall asleep. As a bonus, it doesn't leave you feeling like you're hungover the next morning, as some sleeping pills do, says Varro E. Tyler, Ph.D., distinguished professor emeritus of pharmacognosy at Purdue University in West Lafayette, Indiana. Valerian smells awful, though, so take it in capsule form rather than as a tea. Follow the instructions on the label.

2. Ask questions to live longer. A study funded by the National Institute on Aging followed 1,100 seniors for 5 years and discovered that the most curious of the seniors had a 30 percent better chance of living beyond the 5-year mark than the less inquisitive subjects. According to David Larson, M.D., of the National Institute for Healthcare Research, "Higher curiosity levels may mean better adaptation to changes, stress, or challenges." Another possibility:

Losing your curiosity may signal a life-shortening decline in nervous-system activity.

3. **Do some aerobic exercise for your brain.** Working out will help your body, and according to research, it will also give your brain a boost. Studies have shown that regular aerobic exercise—activities like running and bicycling—can improve your ability to perform more than one task at a time and make you more creative. Doctors aren't entirely sure why this works, but they believe that since exercise improves your cardiovascular system, you may get more blood, oxygen, and nutrients to your brain.

4. **Drink to your memory.** Scientists have found that alcohol may actually boost your memory. According to a study by researchers in the Netherlands, people who have a drink or two a day seem to be half as likely to have poor thinking ability as teetotalers. Further, French researchers found that among 2,273 people over the age of 65, those who drank 8 to 16 ounces of wine a day were much less likely to develop dementia, which may be an early stage of Alzheimer's disease, than people who drank less or no wine.

5. **Take a progressive attitude.** When you're feeling stressed, try this progressive relaxation technique: Alternately tense and relax each part of your body, starting with your toes and working your way up to your scalp. Combine the tensing and releasing with your in/out breathing, suggests Margaret A. Caudill, M.D., Ph.D., co-director of the department of pain medicine at Dartmouth Hitchcock Clinic in Manchester, New Hampshire. For instance, curl the toes on your right foot as you breathe in, then relax them as you breathe out. Then flex your right foot toward your head, breathing in; release, breathing out. Next tense your right leg from the knee downward on the breath in and relax it on the breath out. Then tense your right hip and buttock as you breathe in, relaxing as you breathe out. Move to your left toes and up to your left hip before progressing the rest of the way up your body.

6. **For better mental skills, fuel up with boron.** The micronutrient boron appears to be good for memory, attention, and motor skills, according to James G. Penland, Ph.D., research psychologist at the USDA Grand Forks Human Nutrition Research Center in North Dakota. Research showed that men who consumed 3.25 milligrams of boron each day scored better on tests of all three of those traits than men who ate a low-boron diet. Peanuts are a great source of boron, with 0.5 milligram per ounce. Of course, they're also extremely high in calories and fat. Other foods that give you a boron boost: prunes, dates, and raisins, each with 0.5 milligram per ounce, and honey, with 0.2 milligram per ounce.

7. **Give yourself a break.** Hey, Mr. Negative! Lighten up! Men who think the worst of themselves may be headed for early graves, according to a University of Michigan study. Researchers found that men who saw every personal setback as a catastrophe had a 25 percent greater risk of death and died an average of 2 years earlier than men who addressed their failures more positively.

8. **Don't let urgency be the winning factor.** Too much to do and too little time to do it in? Learn to prioritize. Buy yourself an organizer and actually use it. Plan your days and weeks on paper, listing the priority tasks. Adjust your schedule as needed based on importance and urgency and not just on urgency alone, which is often a temptation. And don't forget to schedule time for some R & R.

9. **Be a smart snacker.** Low blood sugar can intensify emotional stress, irritability, and anxiety, says Jack Groppel, Ph.D., an exercise physiologist and vice president of LGE Performance Systems, Inc. in Orlando, Florida. To keep your blood sugar from sinking, snack on something healthy such as fruit every 2 to 2½ hours between moderate-size meals, he suggests.

10. **Go for ginkgo.** Ginkgo biloba may very well turn out to be man's best friend. (Sorry, Fido.) Not only does the herb seem to help solve erectile difficulties, but it also improves thinking ability. The secret behind ginkgo's powers it that it increases blood flow without affecting blood pressure. It's been shown to help with memory problems, concentration difficulties, depression, and dizziness. For the best results, take it in a 50-to-1 extract, advises Terry Willard, Ph.D., president of the Wild Rose College of Natural Healing in Calgary, Alberta, Canada. That means the label should say that it contains 24 percent flavonoid glycosides—the active ingredient that increases blood flow.

11. **Get a life outside of work.** Everyone knows the importance of having hobbies and other interests outside of work. But sometimes we choose hobbies that are really extensions of our jobs: for example, the computer programmer who designs Web pages at night, or the chef who caters small parties on weekends. Yes, you may be able to advance your career with outside activities, but for your mental health, look for hobbies that are completely removed from your career.

12. **Think in new ways.** Table: Chair. Salt: Pepper. Most of us think in preprogrammed ways. So if you're trying to unleash creativity, compare things that seem to have nothing in common. French fry: B-52 bomber. Fence post: Laptop computer. Take a few minutes to list all of the similarities you can think of between the items. "This helps you make new associations and see things in new ways," says William Shephard, chief of programs for the Creative Education Foundation in Buffalo, New York. "It can break up the thought patterns that most of us always fall into."

Once you're finished with that warm-up, move on to the real problem. If you're trying to think of new ways to market your company's candy bar, compare its attributes to those of the Eiffel Tower. Or Bigfoot. Or the paneling in the conference room. Make a list of the similarities, then see if any of them warrant further discussion.

7

CURES

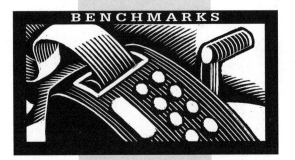

■ Average number of Americans killed each week by prescription drugs: 1,900

■ Average number of different drug prescriptions filled each year by an American over the age of 74: 12

■ Chance that an antidepressant pharmaceutical drug will alleviate severe depression: 1 in 2

■ Chance that a placebo will alleviate severe depression: 1 in 3

■ Ratio of the number of Americans killed in traffic accidents in 1998 to the number killed by medical errors: 1:1

■ Percentage change since 1995 in the number of surgeons worldwide using maggots to cleanse wounds : +400

■ Fee charged by a Pennsylvania cyberpsychologist for online treatment of Internet addiction, per minute: $1.50

■ Estimated number of people who watched a live hair transplant on the Internet: 8,000

■ Percentage of contact lens wearers who say their intimate relationships have improved since they began wearing lenses: 56

■ Percentage of emergency room visits that aren't emergencies: 53

■ Percentage of Americans who say that their doctors have diagnosed a condition or suggested a treatment that turned out to be wrong: 25

■ Number of people who receive some form of professional health care in their home: 2.4 million

■ Number of surgical procedures performed on men annually: 16 million

■ Number of annual office visits men make to physicians: 300 million

■ Number of annual office visits women make to physicians: 471.4 million

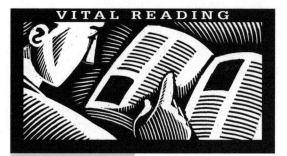

VITAL READING

NFL Secrets for Injury Relief

Use these tips from NFL trainers the next time you get injured playing your favorite weekend sport.

As the head trainer of the Washington Redskins, Bubba Tyer sees more athletic injuries in a week than your family doctor sees in a year. The damage can be gruesome—remember when Lawrence Taylor snapped Joe Theismann's leg like a chicken wing on Monday Night Football?—or it can simply be stupid, like the neck injury that the quarterback Gus Frerotte suffered when he celebrated a touchdown by ramming his head into a wall.

Frerotte is gone from the team, proof that the smart, not necessarily the strong, survive. But Tyer is back for his 29th season with the same goal he's had all along: to help his players recover from injuries as quickly as possible.

So that you can get the same treatment for your assorted injuries, aches, and pains, here is advice from Tyer and his staff as well as David Price, head trainer of the New York Jets.

You twist an ankle rounding third. Once you've finished swearing, grab some ice out of the beer cooler, wrap it in a towel, and put it on your ankle immediately—your recovery time is determined in the first crucial minutes after the injury. If you wait until after the game—or, worse, after the beers after the game—you can double the time you spend on the disabled list.

When you're back home, elevate and wrap the joint. If you don't have an elastic bandage, pull a stretchy dress sock over the ice bag to keep it firmly in place. Keep the ice on for no more than 20 minutes at a time, and wait for the cold feeling to subside before reapplying it.

Best defense: Taping your own ankle is more difficult than upside-down origami, and at $4 a roll, athletic tape is expensive. Instead, protect your gimpy ankle with a lace-up ankle brace. "It'll do as good a job as tape," says Kevin Bastin, a 10-year assistant to Tyer.

You wrench your lower back doing deadlifts. Strains happen frequently to guys who lift weights or play sports in which twisting is involved, such as softball. The key to treating one, Tyer says, is moist heat. The Redskins use heat packs called Hydroculators—compresses that stay warm for up to 15 minutes. You can buy them at drugstores, or you can get the same effect by running a folded towel under warm water and placing it on the affected area. Reheat as needed.

Best defense: Some lower-back pain is caused by an imbalance between strong back muscles and weak abdominal muscles. To fix the problem, work on your gut. Sets of 20 crunches are a good start, says Price.

Your body aches after a tough workout. If you played sports in high school, you remember the soothing relief of Ben-Gay on sore muscles (and the burning when that locker-room funnyman applied it to your jockstrap). The Redskins use two similar products, Flexall and Tiger Balm, to help loosen stiff muscles and balky joints. Squeeze a dab into your hand and massage it into the muscle with your fingers. "It can heat up the area and make it more comfortable," says Tyer. "And the massage increases blood flow. That helps muscles heal more quickly." Makes you smell like an athlete, too.

Best defense: Don't take tomorrow off. NFL teams play on Sundays, but their day off is Tuesday. The reason is that waste products, such as lactic acid, build up in muscles after intense work. If left to sit, they harden, making you even more sore 2 days after your game. By doing a light workout the day after a tough one, you can move the junk out of your muscles earlier and recover faster.

You get the wind knocked out of you. Try to relax as you wait to regain your breath—panicking can lead to hyperventilation when your lungs finally start working again. When you're able, clamber to your knees and breathe in through your nose and out through your mouth.

You jam your finger catching a pass. Ice it immediately to prevent swelling. If the pain and stiffness persist for more than a few hours, have an x-ray. Unless there's a break or severe ligament damage, your biggest problem will be scar tissue, which can lead to gnarled knuckles, says Tyer. To hinder scar-tissue formation, don't splint the finger, and keep it moving as much as possible.

Best defense: If you have a digit that is frequently jammed, try buddy-taping it to a neighboring finger, suggests Tyer. Two fingers are stronger than one, and less likely to bend at an odd angle.

You wake up with a crick in your neck. Take ibuprofen for the pain and swelling, then hop into a warm shower and angle the spray to hit the sore area. After a few minutes, gently roll your neck back and forth like a boxer to loosen up the muscles. You can try to exercise, but don't do anything that makes the pain worse. If it doesn't feel better in a day or so, see your doctor.

You're kicked in the balls. Sit down and put your head between your legs. This will help stop that sick feeling in the pit of your stomach, says Price. Next, reach into your shorts and count your little buddies. If there's only one, his partner may have been knocked up into your abdomen. You'll need to see your doctor to coax it back down. You'll also need to see a doc if there's swelling, bruising, or prolonged pain. Ice the injured gonad on your way to the physician. The cold will be intense, so apply it over your underwear.

You fall off your bike and skin your elbow. Injuries like this aren't deep, but the large surface area makes them more likely than regular gashes to become infected. Be extra-vigilant if you receive your wound by falling or diving on artificial turf—fake grass harbors a lot of bacteria, says Al Bellamy, an assistant trainer with the Redskins. Wash the abrasion thoroughly and keep it covered.

That 240-pound power forward elbows you in the face. Pinch your schnozz to stanch the flow of blood, and lean your head back. Put a bag of ice on the bridge of your nose. The cold will help stop the bleeding even faster. Don't return to the game right away; ask one of the cheerleaders for a tampon, cut off a piece, and use it to plug your nostril. "They are extra-absorbent," says Price. And you'll feel "extra-fresh."

You take a puck in the teeth. A dentist can reimplant a knocked-out tooth, but you have to get to his chair within 30 minutes. Before you hop in the car, clean the tooth with water and store it in a cup of milk.

Best defense: If you're playing a contact sport, wear a mouthguard. It protects you against losing teeth and can lower your chances of a jaw fracture or concussion by acting as a shock absorber, Tyer says. Your dentist can fit you with an extra-thin one that's hardly noticeable.

You pull a hamstring legging out an infield single. Fill a paper cup with water and stick it in your freezer. Next time you abuse a muscle, tear off the top half of the cup, put a paper towel over the ice, and rub it over the damaged tissue. This will push swelling out, speeding recovery. Applying the ice while gently stretching the muscle seems to help even more, Tyer says.

Best defense: To loosen up, jog or hit the exercise bike for 10 minutes before practice or a competition. If you play softball or another sport in which you cool off between bursts of activity, continue to stretch and jog even when out of the action.

Your opponent bites you. In the heat of competition, just about anything can happen. (Conrad Dobler, the former St. Louis Cardinals lineman, is said to have toothed a number of defensive tackles.) If some idiot decides to take a chunk out of your leg at the bottom of a scrum, go to your doctor immediately. "Human bites are deadly serious because of the high risk of infection and disease," Price says. "No matter how superficial a bite is, you need to see a professional."

You get beaned in the head. If a shot to the melon makes you dizzy or nauseated, stop what you're doing immediately and have someone take you to see a doctor. "Being disoriented or having blurred vision are also signs you need medical attention," Price says. Be wary of symptoms even hours after the blow, and avoid taking aspirin or ibuprofen for pain; they can encourage hemorrhaging. Take Tylenol instead.

You tear a rotator cuff. Trying to gun a guy out at the plate after a winter of channel surfing is a great way to injure your rotator cuff, which can take months to heal. A tear usually shows up as vague pain in the shoulder area, and it may result in a "catching" sensation when the arm is rotated. See your doctor if a day or two of reduced activity doesn't help. The initial treatment is rest and anti-inflammatories. But as soon as pain levels permit, start physical therapy to regain motion.

Best defense: Do lateral and front raises with 5-pound dumbbells to strengthen the smaller muscles in your shoulder. Also, Price says, you should stretch your shoulder joint frequently by draping a towel over your shoulder, grasping it with the opposite hand, and pulling it up and down, as if you were drying your back. Do 10 repetitions on each shoulder. If you play softball, warm up between innings to keep loose.

You dislocate a shoulder. If one of your shoulders pops out of joint, you'll be able to tell by its appearance and by your bloodcurdling screams. If this is a repeat dislocation, you may be able to gently coax it back into the joint yourself. Don't try to do a Mel Gibson and force it back; you might do even more damage to the ligaments.

A separated shoulder is essentially a sprain, and should be treated with ice and anti-inflammatories and a trip to the doctor. Tip: Because of your shoulder's shape, it can be difficult to make a bag of ice cubes stay in contact with the joint. Instead of cubes, try crushed or flaked ice. With a little pressure, it will form to your shoulder, providing even, constant cold.

You're smacked in the eye with a squash ball. Any injury to your eyes warrants careful evaluation by a doctor, says Price. Be especially concerned if your vision is distorted. If you take a blow to the eye, you can put an ice pack over your eye socket, but it's smart to keep it off your eyelid.

If a foreign object enters your eye, wash it away immediately by flushing the eye with eyewash (or water, in a pinch). Even a speck of dirt can cause infection or a scratch on your cornea. If it lodges under a contact lens, it can cause an ulceration. "Always stop what you're doing and rinse away anything that gets in your eye," Price says.

You take an elbow to the ribs. Your ribs are involved in every activity you enjoy, especially breathing. Use a cold compress for mild discomfort. "If serious pain persists for more than a day, or gets worse, you should see your doctor," Price says. But expect even mild rib-cartilage damage to take a month or so to clear up.

Stomp Out Sinusitis

If you have cold symptoms that just won't go away, it could be sinusitis. Try these easy tips for relief.

Your latest cold, the one that's been plaguing you for weeks, may have come from an unlikely source: that bad-hop grounder that broke your nose 23 years ago.

A broken nose, a deviated septum, or any other quirk that prevents your sinuses from draining properly—even a cold—can cause sinusitis, an inflammation brought on by bacterial infection.

About 35 million Americans are suffering from sinusitis right now. It may have struck you dozens of times: Your sinus passages become swollen during a cold or allergy attack, trapping mucus filled with bacteria, which soon infect your sinus tissue. You stay pitifully sick for at least 3 weeks, three times as long as most colds last.

Of course, you always mistake sinusitis for a cold. That's because most symptoms are identical: sinus pain, headaches, congestion. But there's one foolproof sign: Sinusitis doesn't cause sneezing. What it does cause is thick yellow mucus; colds and allergies, on the other hand, usually produce thin, pale-colored mucus. That's why your doctor is always inquiring after the state of your phlegm.

You can't prevent sinusitis, but you'd better treat it fast, says Wellington Tichenor, M.D., a New York allergist. The longer your sinuses remain infected, the more vulnerable they are to repeated infections, and that can make them permanently swollen. If this occurs, you'll wheeze through life feeling punkier than Iggy Pop. If cold symptoms ever persist longer than 10 days, see your doctor. You might need a 2-week course of antibiotics to fight sinusitis. The following tips also help relieve the misery.

Get the hell up. Sinusitis symptoms are worst in the morning, because mucus pools in your head overnight. In fact, lying down for just 30 minutes can increase your nasal congestion by 20 percent. So set the alarm.

Take a long, steaming shower. Invite a friend, too. Steam helps shrink your swollen sinuses, and sex stops you from caring.

Eat grapefruit. It's the best source of glutathione, an antioxidant that may help regulate sinus pressure. A study from the Netherlands found that people with chronic sinusitis had lower levels of glutathione in their nasal linings than healthy subjects did. Oranges, peaches, asparagus, potatoes, and broccoli are also good sources.

Dilute your decongestant. If you take a medicated nasal decongestant, like Afrin, don't overdo it. Using it for just 3 days in a row can irritate your nasal lining and make sinusitis worse, says Alexander C. Chester, M.D., of Georgetown University in Washington, D.C. To prevent this, replace half of your decongestant spray with water that's been boiled for 10 minutes. This diluted solution should still relieve symptoms well, and you can use it for up to 6 days.

Sweat at lunch. "Vigorous exercise can clear sinuses almost as well as taking Sudafed," says Dr. Chester. "That's because adrenaline acts as a vasoconstrictor—it shrinks swollen membranes in your nose."

Go heavy on the horseradish. The hot spread contains allyl isothiocyanate, a nasal-clearing chemical used in some decongestants, says Sanford Archer, M.D., of the University of Kentucky Medical Center in Lexington. At home, sniff a jar of horseradish as a booster shot—unless it expired in 9/95.

Snort a salt spray. It constricts swollen nasal tissues, says Dr. Tichenor. Use a nonmedicated saline spray, such as NaSal or AYR Saline Nasal Mist. Or, if you're cheap, throw a teaspoon of salt into 2 cups of water that has been boiled for 10 minutes, pour some in a shot glass, and snort a bit up one nostril at a time. You'll probably gag, so put away the photo album first.

Be a light-beer weenie. Lay off heavy stouts and ales at happy hour; they contain molds that can aggravate sinusitis, says Dr. Chester. That's partly why your face often feels "puffy" after you sling back a few dark imports. The higher alcohol content can also thicken mucus by dehydrating you. "If you drink, you're better off having a lighter beer like Miller or Coors Light," he says. One vice you can't afford is smoking. Inhaling smoke makes mucus thicker and aggravates sinusitis, explains Dr. Chester.

Eat chicken soup—on steroids. For a truly sinus-blasting meal, sprinkle ½ teaspoon of cayenne pepper and ½ teaspoon of garlic powder into chicken soup. The spicy pepper and garlic slightly irritate your nasal passages, which helps them expand so you can breathe more easily. Chicken contains cysteine, an amino acid that relieves mucus buildup and a scratchy throat.

Uncork the chardonnay. Don't drink red wine; it contains some substance (quite possibly the tannins) that swells your sinus tissues, says Dr. Chester. He found that 28 percent of his patients had worse sinusitis symptoms after drinking red wine.

Do the "secret squirrel" trick. Before you drift off, rub your sinuses by pressing your thumbs on both sides of your nose for 30 seconds, several times. This will increase blood flow and help relieve the sinus aches you feel when lying down.

If you suffer repeated bouts of sinusitis that antibiotics can't cure, you need to have x-rays to determine what's blocking your sinuses, says Dr. Archer. You might need endoscopic surgery to breathe freely. In an outpatient procedure, a surgeon can enlarge your sinus openings so future infections won't close them entirely. It's a last resort, though, because full recovery can take months and there have been rare complications.

When Your Heart Skips a Beat

Here are eight harmless things that could be affecting your heart.

You spend your whole life listening to your heart. It's got a great beat, and you can dance to it. But when it skips, it's amazing how fast you can assume the worst—that the slightest twinge means a toe tag to follow shortly. True, if your rhythm is out of whack or if you have heart pain, you should have it checked out. But not every heart hiccup means you'll soon be walking toward the light. In fact, a number of (nonfatal) circumstances might cause your heart to thump like a '72 Chevy with 16-inch woofers. For instance, it could be any of the following factors.

A can of Coke. Temporary heart palpitations—a condition called supraventricular tachycardia—are enough to scare the hell out of you, but sudden rapid heartbeats are usually harmless. Often they're triggered by caffeine or nicotine, which means you can eliminate the palpitations by cutting out the vice that's causing them, says Paul Mahoney, M.D., of the University of Pennsylvania's Health Center in Philadelphia. If pain or dizziness accompanies irregular beats, or if they last more than a few seconds, see a doctor to rule out more serious stuff.

The company party. After a big night out, quickening palpitations could signal a common condition known as holiday-heart syndrome, so named because it often coincides with raucous Christmas parties. Drinking a lot of booze can lead to a machine gun–like pulse. "We usually see it when people suddenly drink way more than usual on one particular night or over a weekend," says David Hayes, M.D., a cardiologist at the Mayo Clinic. People don't normally die from it, but they do get fired.

Constipation. It's a classic heart-attack symptom—fainting, that is. But just because you keel over doesn't mean you're dying. Fainting is often caused by dehydration, strenuous coughing, or—from the Pray-This-Never-Happens-to-You category—a bowel movement. "Straining can alter the pressure in your chest and reduce the blood flow to your head, so you faint," says Dr. Hayes. If you feel you're going to faint during physical exertion, however, stop what you're doing and get someone to take you to an emergency room. Abnormal heart rhythms require immediate attention. Just ask any Celtics fan.

Your personal-best bench press. While the pain from a heart attack feels as if someone were tightening a belt around your chest, the pain from a muscle pull or strain feels sharp and knifelike, says Jonathan Zaroff, M.D., a cardiologist at the University of California at San Francisco. Try raising or lowering your arms to see if that helps alleviate the pain. If it does, stay off the weights for a few days. If it doesn't, call 911—just to be on the safe side.

A small leak. That small flutter you feel is just a defect in one of your heart valves. Sounds serious, we know. Actually, it's probably innocuous: A valve simply isn't opening and closing as efficiently as it should. The skipped beat, or heart murmur, could be the blood trying to pass through that malfunctioning valve. If you have a murmur, you may need antibiotics before surgery or dental work. Bacteria can easily pool around a malfunctioning valve, putting you at risk for infections.

Those six burrito supremes. Men often think they're having heart attacks when what they really have is just a bad case of indigestion or heartburn. An antacid should relieve the burning sensation in a few minutes, says Dr. Zaroff. If it doesn't, do a self-check for other classic heart-attack symptoms, such as dizziness, sweating, and pain in your jaw.

A bug. Any viral infection that causes flulike symptoms can also lead to inflammation of the heart, says Douglas Zipes, M.D., of the Indiana University School of Medicine in Indianapolis. Inflamed heart tissue can disrupt the flow of the tiny electrical current that causes the heart to beat. When the infection leaves, so do the irregular heartbeats. If they don't, see a doctor.

Your in-laws. Chest pain and irregular heartbeats can signal anxiety or extreme stress. Antianxiety drugs may help; so might moving 2,000 miles away.

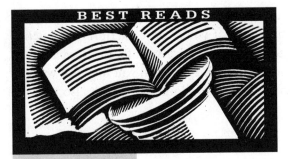

BEST READS

Three Herbs for a Healthy Prostate

If you've been diagnosed with benign prostatic hyperplasia (BPH), you've likely been prescribed a synthetic medication, often Flomax or Proscar. Yet some experts believe that herbs can treat the condition just as effectively as drugs—and herbs offer fewer side effects and are easier on the wallet. In the following excerpt from Natural Prostate Healers: A Breakthrough Program for Preventing and Treating Common Prostate Problems *(Prentice Hall), author Mike Fillon discusses three herbs—saw palmetto, pygeum, and stinging nettles—that offer promise for men who already have BPH or who want to prevent it in the first place.*

Herbs have been used as medicines for thousands of years. In fact, many of the pharmaceutical products sold today are synthetic chemicals based on herbal extracts. Herbal medicines may contain a whole plant, parts of a plant, or extracts of either one or a combination of plants.

Many people prefer to use herbal medicines because in many cases they exert beneficial effects without the side effects caused by many pharmaceutical drugs, such as prostate drugs.

Doctors often prescribe two aggressively marketed drugs for benign prostatic hyperplasia (BPH), including terazosin HCI (Abbott Laboratories' Hytrin) or finasteride (Merck and Company's Proscar). Unfortunately, their side effects include dizziness, impotence, and loss of libido.

Herbs have played a significant role in BPH treatment for years. Specifically, alternative practitioners have recommended three safe, effective, and inexpensive herbs for the treatment of BPH: saw palmetto (*Serenoa repens*), pygeum (*Pygeum africanum*), and stinging nettles (*Urtica dioica*). Their value in BPH has been documented in European medical journals since the early 1970s, long before they were approved for use in the United States. These three herbs, along with pumpkin seed oil and pollen, have resulted in a drop in surgery rates for BPH and a safer, more cost-efficient approach for managing the condition. Moreover, there's evidence they can fight prostatitis and even prostate cancer.

Before you take any of the supplements mentioned here, I recommend you check with your doctor first, especially if you're on prescription medicine. There may be a conflict. Also, sometimes botanicals conflict with each other. For example, if you're on blood thinning medication, you may not want to take garlic or the memory enhancer ginkgo biloba, since both also thin the blood.

Native American Healers Were Right

Long ago, Native American men knew that the dark, brownish-black berries from a small palm tree that grew wild in Florida, Georgia, Louisiana, and South Carolina were an effective cure for "male problems." Then during the early part of this century, a tea made from saw palmetto berries was commonly recommended in the United States for prostate and urinary tract problems. It was also thought to increase sperm production and sex drive in men and became a popular male tonic. As a result, saw palmetto has been recognized by the United States Pharmacopoeia as a remedy for prostate problems since 1905.

Research in Europe in the 1960s led to the discovery of the oil portion of the berry and its medically active free fatty acids, ethyl esters, and sterols. Today, the extract is considered natural, safe, and inexpensive, and it has no known side effects in treating BPH.

Saw palmetto attacks BPH from several fronts. The enzyme 5-AR is believed to be the culprit that speeds up the conversion of testosterone to dihydrotestosterone (DHT) as men age. This increased 5-AR activity and subsequent increases in prostate levels of DHT appear to have a major influence on the formation of BPH. The saw palmetto berries contain substances that actively inhibit the enzyme from making this conversion.

But that's not all. Other hormones may also contribute to formation of BPH, including estrogen, progesterone, and prolactin. Saw palmetto reduces the effects of estrogen and progesterone on the prostate. It also "cools" inflammation in the gland itself and inhibits the formation of inflammatory substances that contribute to increasing the size of the prostate and can lead to prostatitis. Since high levels of DHT also correlate with prostate cancer, saw palmetto may also help prevent this disease.

Men suffering with BPH are generally offered drug therapy to control it in its earlier stages. As I've said, prescription prostate drugs have serious side effects, including impotence. When compared to finasteride, the drug most commonly prescribed for BPH, the saw palmetto extract consistently shows higher effectiveness in improving prostate symptoms, with far fewer side effects. Saw palmetto works the same way finasteride does—it prevents the breakdown of testosterone to dihydrotestosterone. Plus, studies show this herb to be remarkably safe.

In 1984, Dr. G. Champault, a well-known British scientist, conducted one of the first double-blind studies to show that saw palmetto actually counteracts the hormonal imbalances that are the most common cause of prostate enlargement. The results of Dr. Champault's study were so impressive that he excited the interest of the medical community. As a result, numerous prominent scientists at nine medical research centers around Europe decided to conduct their own double-blind studies on the saw palmetto extract.

Since the mid-1980s, at least 10 studies on more than 1,000 patients in Europe have confirmed the value of saw palmetto. Specifically, an amazing 90 percent of the patients who were given this extract experienced remarkable relief from their symptoms.

If you're the type of guy who needs proof, here are summaries of many of the studies performed on saw palmetto. Me? I like to know as much as possible about something before I start gulping it down. I want to know if I'm creating a whole new slew of problems, or if I'm just producing expensive urine.

However, if you're a trusting soul, or numbers bore you, you're not going to hurt my feelings by skipping over the numbers. But if you decide to do that, make sure you don't miss the important stuff.

That said, here's a quick summary of saw palmetto research.

• German studies of up to 200 men with BPH, as well as those in British, French, and Italian medical journals, have confirmed the value of saw palmetto extract. The dose of extracts in the studies typically was 320 milligrams per day, in two divided doses.

• A 1-year study in Hungary found that 320 milligrams of saw palmetto extract daily led to a reduction in residual urine (the urine left in the bladder after urination) and an increase in urinary flow rates. These results were considered significant by the sixth month of treatment.

• One 28-day study with 110 BPH patients found 320 milligrams per day was effective in reducing painful urination, nighttime urination, and urine residue left in the bladder. There was also a significant improvement in urine flow rate. Forty-seven patients were then followed for 15 to 30 months and were found to have continued improvement.

• In another study, researchers followed 305 BPH patients who took 160 milligrams of saw palmetto extract twice daily. At the end of 90 days, 88 percent of the patients rated the treatment a success. Their physicians' evaluations were equally favorable. Urinary flow rate improved significantly and there was a notable decrease in prostate size.

In one recent 3-month study, 88 percent of the patients treated with saw palmetto and their physicians reported:
- Improvement in urinary flow
- Less residual urine
- Reduced prostate size

Other results noted included:
- Fewer nighttime visits to the bathroom
- (Ahh!) A stronger stream

Not surprisingly, there is currently a huge market in Europe for saw palmetto. Guess what? Its popularity in the United States is growing by leaps and bounds, too.

So here's a summary of the good news about saw palmetto.
- Besides being effective and free of side effects, saw palmetto costs about one-third as much as prostate medications such as Proscar.
- Men who take saw palmetto for BPH usually notice results after 2 to 6 weeks, though most use the herb longer for more complete relief.
- Many doctors are learning that saw palmetto is an inexpensive and safe way to maintain prostate health. For younger men, this herb can help prevent prostate problems later on in life.

In order for saw palmetto to be effective, it must be in an extract form (usually capsules, though tinctures are also used). Since the active ingredients are fat soluble, a tea made from the berries would not give much benefit.

Dr. Julian Whitaker, who practices alternative medicine in Potomac, Maryland, says to prevent BPH, men should start taking saw palmetto extract on a regular basis in their mid-forties. For those who do not yet have a problem, he recommends a dosage of 80 milligrams twice a day. For those who already have a prostate problem, he recommends taking 160 to 320 milligrams of the extract each day while under the watchful eye of a physician. He also says such men should have a urine flow check every 30 to 60 days.

Out of Africa, a Natural Cure for Prostate Disorders

High in the mountains of central and southern Africa, the bark of a large evergreen tree yields another herb that decreases prostate swelling. In fact, the powdered bark from *Pygeum africanum* has been used by locals as a tea for relief of urinary disorders for ages.

European scientists exploring traditional herbal medicines were so impressed with reports of pygeum's actions that they began laboratory investigations. As was the case with saw palmetto, this led to the development of an extract of the bark. As a result, it's been used extensively in France and elsewhere in Europe, and recently has been imported into the United States.

Now, you may be asking, how do they discover these things? Who's the brave soul who first peels off the bark, tastes it and discovers it's a remedy for some ailment? I don't know. I'm just glad someone did.

Pygeum seems to work, like saw palmetto, by limiting the formation of DHT. It also lowers prolactin levels, a pituitary hormone related to prostate and sexual function. Pygeum has additionally proven useful for the treatment of chronic, non-bacterial prostatitis, a condition that leads to inflammation of the prostate and can affect males at any age.

In 1997, in the British medical journal *Lancet*, German researchers reported on a study of 200 men who had symptoms due to BPH. Half received a placebo and half 60 milligrams per day of beta-sitosterol, which is one of the main active ingredients extracted from *Pygeum africanum* bark. It or similar compounds are also present in other herbs that are used to treat the prostate.

After three months, the men taking beta-sitosterol extract had a statistically significant improvement in the velocity of urine flow. Those taking the placebo did not.

Scientists are not exactly sure how beta-sitosterol works to improve prostate symptoms. One interesting tie-in is that it lowers blood cholesterol. It's believed that accumulation of cholesterol in the prostate increases the binding sites for testosterone and DHT. These researchers are also convinced high cholesterol is an important factor stimulating prostate growth. Another good reason to watch your diet!

Here's a summary of other research on pygeum.

- In several double-blind studies, a fat-soluble extract of this herb improved prostate symptoms significantly without many side effects (of these, stomach irritation was the most common). In fact, in one study, sexual ability was increased as well. So, besides helping relieve BPH symptoms (and sexual disorders due to BPH), pygeum may work for those with prostatitis.
- Pygeum extract (100 milligrams per day) or a placebo was administered to 263 BPH patients for 60 days. The pygeum group showed marked clinical improvement, with noticeable increase in urinary flow rate.
- Eighteen patients with either BPH or chronic prostatitis were treated with pygeum (200 milligrams per day) for 60 days. Urination performance parameters improved and there was a measured reduction in prostate size in BPH patients as well as reduced inflammation in the prostatitis patients.

- Twenty BPH patients, ages 51 to 89, were given either pygeum (200 milligrams per day) or a placebo for 60 days. Again, the pygeum group showed a significantly greater improvement of BPH symptoms.
- An Italian study published in 1991 reported that not only did pygeum reduce urinary problems and prostate inflammation, but it also increased sexual desire. La dolce vita!

Take the Sting Out of Pain

Another herbal treatment for BPH is the root of stinging nettles (*Urtica dioica*). Stinging nettles, which can grow just about anywhere, have little prickly hairs that stick in your skin and sting and itch like crazy (thus their name). Aside from the stinging factor, the nettle is a very useful plant. It is edible and contains minerals such as iron, silica, potassium, manganese, and sulfur, as well as vitamins A and C. It also has many medicinal applications.

The fresh green leaves may be cooked and eaten like spinach, or made into soup or tea. (Fortunately, the sting is not present in the cooked or dried plant form.) A tea made from the leaves is a powerful tonic that provides many important vitamins and minerals. The vitamin C content works to help the iron be absorbed by the body. There are many folk and homeopathic medicinal uses for nettles, including stopping BPH. Like saw palmetto and pygeum, it blocks the formation of DHT.

There's been a limited number of double-blind studies supporting its effectiveness for use with prostate problems. One study of 67 men with BPH found that supplements of this herb reduced nighttime urination. A typical dose is 300 milligrams of an extract.

If these three herbs are so good, would taking more than one of them supergalvanize your prostate? As you might expect, some researchers say combinations of at least two of these herbs exert greater benefits at low doses.

Two recent studies looked at a combination of saw palmetto extract and nettle root to treat BPH. They were impressive because of the large number of patients followed in the first study, and the head-to-head comparison with Proscar in the second.

The first study followed 2,080 BPH patients for 12 weeks. Men in the study were treated with a combination of saw palmetto extract (160 milligrams) and nettle root extract (120 milligrams) twice daily. The saw palmetto/nettle root combination produced:

- 26 percent increase in maximum urinary flow
- 44.7 percent reduction in residual urine
- 62.5 percent reduction in painful urination

• 53.6 percent reduction in post-urination dribbling

• 50 percent reduction in nighttime urination

A recent 1-year study comparing the saw palmetto and nettle root combination versus Proscar showed equal improvement in both groups after 6 months of treatment.

A French research study noted that a combination therapy of stinging nettles and pygeum led to dramatic improvements in BPH in only 1 month. Likewise, a combination of saw palmetto and nettle root has been the focus of two important clinical studies. Several studies have also shown that saw palmetto and *Pygeum africanum* work well together.

It's up to you to decide if you want to take more than one. Remember, they all work well on their own. I've been taking 160 milligrams of saw palmetto every day for about 18 months. I'm happy to report my doctor told me I have had no prostate enlargement. Also, my stream and libido are just fine, thank you. (Knock on wood!)

However, if you're the type who believes two or more are better than one—and money is no object—go ahead. I do recommend, though, you start with just one. If you show no negative response, such as stomach problems, add another.

Saw palmetto, pygeum, and stinging nettles extracts offer a safe and cost-effective approach to men with BPH or those who want to prevent it in the first place. Medical experts say patients using the first two usually begin showing effects within 3 to 4 weeks of use. However, men who already have BPH will need to continue use for at least 6 to 9 months to determine true effectiveness.

Once you're convinced they work, doctors say you will need to incorporate either saw palmetto, pygeum, or nettles into your daily supplement routine for the long term since many patients have noted a return of symptoms within 1 or 2 weeks of stopping any of the extracts. Face it, it's going to become part of your daily regimen. It's a good thing the herbs are considerably cheaper than the drugs they mimic.

You'll be able to find saw palmetto more easily than the other two. I've seen it in drug, food, discount, and convenience stores, while I've seen pygeum and nettles only in health food and vitamin stores.

First-Aid for Your Back Attack

If you own a pickup truck, you already know that you're Mr. Popular when friends, family—heck, even acquaintances—are moving. Sure, you may get a few brews out of the deal, but that's hardly a fair trade-off for the backache you're likely to feel the next day. In the following chapter from Back Pain Remedies for Dummies *(IDG Books Worldwide), authors Michael S. Sinel, M.D., and William W.*

Deardorff, Ph.D., offer some home remedies to fight the pain and get you back on your feet.

So, things seem to be going along relatively smoothly. You have your job, you have your family, and you make time to have a little fun. Then, like a blind-sided tackle in a football game, the back attack hits. Your back attack may consist of a slight pain and stiffness in your lower back area. Or the pain may significantly restrict your movements and cause you distress. You may even have pain running down one or both legs.

Perhaps you have just hit the perfect drive on the eighth hole of your favorite golf course. Maybe you lifted a heavy piece of equipment at work. Maybe you bent over to pick up a pencil. Or, maybe you just woke up with back pain one morning. In any case, the back pain hit and got your attention in a major way.

Fortunately, all is not lost (not even close!). Whatever your situation, you can choose from several techniques—which we discuss in this chapter—to help you manage your back attack successfully.

Heading for the Doctor

You can manage and treat most episodes of back pain on your own. But, you also need to recognize a few warning signs that mean you should skip the home remedies and head straight to the doctor for an evaluation.

You can't control your bowel or bladder. If you suddenly lose control of your bowel or bladder, you should either see a physician who specializes in spinal problems or go to the emergency room *immediately*. Bowel or bladder problems include the following:

• You can't control or initiate urination or bowel movements
• You have no feeling in your groin and/or anal area
• You can no longer get an erection

Any of the preceding symptoms indicate possible *cauda equina syndrome*. In cauda equina syndrome, some of the nerves that control bowel, bladder, and other functions become compressed. If this compression isn't corrected surgically within about 24 to 48 hours, these problems may become permanent due to nerve damage.

Your legs are weak or you experience foot drop. If you experience weakness in your legs and feet, then you should see a spinal specialist within 24 hours or go to the emergency room. Weakness that occurs in your foot is called foot drop because you have trouble flexing your foot and toes up toward your head. You also have trouble walking because your foot is weak and has a tendency to drag.

Your back pain awakens you at night. Back pain that awakens you from sleep at night can indicate a tumor or spinal infection. This type of pain is called rest pain and involves severe throbbing and aching that worsens with rest. Although many people with back pain report being awakened at night by pain, this pain is different from the constant throbbing that a tumor or spinal infection causes. Although a tumor or spinal infection may not be quite the emergency that cauda equina syndrome can be, you should still see a specialist fairly quickly or go to the emergency room.

You experience a significant trauma such as a car accident or a fall. In general, if you suffer a significant trauma such as a car accident or fall that causes back pain, you should see a doctor. Depending on how bad the pain is, you may go to the emergency room, see your family doctor, or see a spinal specialist. Although most back pain doesn't require imaging studies, your doctor may recommend an x-ray or other imaging test to check for fractured vertebrae if you've had a trauma.

Your back pain is excruciating. If your back pain is simply excruciating and unbearable, then you need to go to the emergency room or to your doctor immediately. Also, a physician should check any significant increase in pain to an excruciating level right away. "Excruciating" is a subjective term; however, if your pain is so bad that you can barely move or are on the verge of tears, don't be a tough guy—have it checked out.

Using Home Remedies

The following home remedy techniques can help you manage your own back pain in the initial stages or during a back pain flare-up. Keep the warning symptoms we discussed in mind when determining whether you need to see a physician.

If your back pain appears to be worsening as you use any of the home remedies, visit your physician or spine specialist.

Other home remedy treatments you may consider include wearing a brace or corset, applying a topical anti-irritant to sore muscles (Ben-Gay or Sports Cream, for example), having your muscles lightly massaged and stretched, and engaging in deep breathing and other relaxation exercises. Always avoid placing direct pressure on or over the spine.

Climb into Bed—But Not for Too Long

In the early stages of back pain or during a significant flare-up in your chronic back pain, the pain may be signaling you that something is wrong—perhaps you're having a muscle spasm, sprain-strain, or something else.

The best course in the early stages of back pain is to let pain be your guide. In other words, listen to the pain signal and stop what you're doing. For instance, if you're in the middle of a sporting activity, you may want to call it a day after doing some cooling down movements such as stretching or gentle walking. Or, if you're at work, you may want to tell your supervisor and either take a break or head home for the remainder of the day. Your response to the pain you're experiencing depends on the degree of the pain. For the sake of this discussion, we assume that your pain is fairly severe, requiring you to stop your activity and go home to bed.

In the old days (about 10 years ago!) doctors recommended weeks of strict bed rest for a back pain problem. The idea was to rest your back until the pain resolved. That thinking has changed, and bed rest is considered one of the worst things you can do. Limit your overall bed rest to about 2 or 3 days. (Up to 5 days maximum of rest may be appropriate in some cases.)

Extended bed rest for back pain promotes muscle weakness, decreased flexibility, stomach and bowel problems, and ultimately, an overall increase in your pain. You can avoid these negative aspects of too much rest by staying somewhat active even in the initial stages of back pain. For instance, in the first day or two of a back attack, you may only be able to walk from your bed to the bathroom and back. Shortly thereafter, though, try to increase your out-of-bed time and walk some more, even if you just walk around the house. Expand this activity as you feel able or as your doctor guides you.

Resting the Right Way

Getting bed rest for your back pain isn't as straightforward as it sounds. You should still feel free to get up occasionally to go to the bathroom and take a lap or two around your home. In fact, you should try to get some movement at least two to four times per day.

You may be tempted while resting in bed (possibly due to significant boredom) to prop yourself up on some pillows and either watch TV or read. However, propping yourself up actually causes more pressure on your discs than if you are standing.

You can assume two optimal positions for your painful back when you're in bed:

• Lie on your side and bend at your hips and knees to 90 degrees. Place a small pillow between your knees.
• Lie on your back with your legs elevated by pillows placed underneath your knees. In this position your hips and knees are bent, and the stress and pressure on your spine is at a minimum.

If you're like some people, you may be more comfortable sleeping on your stomach. Unfortunately, sleeping on your stomach places your spine in a slightly extended position that can cause more pain. If you can't avoid sleeping on your stomach, consider placing a pillow or a towel under your stomach to straighten out your spine. Doing so can help relieve the pressure on your spine if you just can't sleep in any other position.

Getting Out of Bed

You may need a special technique to help you get in and out of the bed without significantly increasing your back pain.

1. Lie on your side while facing the side of the bed from which you plan to get out.
2. While lying on your side, work your way to the edge of the bed, taking care not to fall out of bed and onto the floor.
3. While keeping your back straight, use your lower arm and then the palm of your hand to push yourself slowly up to a sitting position. As you push yourself up, allow your legs to fall over the bed and gently to the floor. You should now be in a sitting position on the bed with your feet planted firmly on the floor.
4. From this position, you can make a smooth transition from the sitting to the standing position. If you have trouble going from the sitting to the standing position, you may want to hold on to the headboard or other stable piece of furniture (such as a dresser or nightstand) while you stand up. If you feel weak or unsafe going from sitting to standing on your own, have someone help you or use an assisting device (a walker or cane) per your doctor's recommendation. Try to do this entire movement without twisting or bending your spine. Keeping your abdominal and gluteal (buttocks) muscles tight can help you safely perform this movement.

To get into bed, simply follow the preceding steps in reverse. Remember to move slowly and smoothly.

After about 2 or 3 days of bed rest, try to increase your level of activity. You may want to try more walking or being up and out of bed for more time during the day. You should also try some gentle knee to chest stretches. To increase movement, you may also want to try doing some other special back exercises. (Your doctor can probably recommend some for you.) If your back pain is so severe that you don't feel that you can increase your movement after about 2 or 3 days of bed rest, consult your physician if you haven't already done so.

Cool Down and Heat Up

Ice and/or heat can go a long way in relieving your back pain, but you should understand how and why they work.

- Ice reduces inflammation initially (due to decreasing blood flow from constricted blood vessels) and provides pain relief.
- Heat causes blood vessels to expand, allowing more blood to flow to the affected area, thereby encouraging healing.

You have a number of ways to apply ice and heat to your back pain. For instance, you can place ice cubes in a plastic bag and then place that in a towel; you can use an ice pack purchased over-the-counter from a drugstore; or you can try using a bag of frozen peas.

Never apply ice directly to your skin for more than five minutes at a time because it can freeze the skin and cause soft-tissue damage. If the ice isn't directly on the skin or is not making you uncomfortable, then apply ice for up to 20 minutes every 2 hours.

You can also apply heat in a number of different ways. For instance, you can heat a moist towel in the microwave, use a heating pad, or select from a variety of moist heating pads at your drugstore.

Don't make your towel or heating pad so hot that you risk burning your skin or that it makes you uncomfortable.

One of the most common questions patients ask us is when to apply cold and when to apply heat. Take a look at two common tenets about when to apply ice and heat:

- Most doctors say to apply ice or heat as feels best for you. This decision may include predominantly one or the other, whichever seems to provide the most benefit for you. Also, you can alternate ice and heat.
- Other doctors recommend ice in the first 48 hours after the injury and then heat thereafter. The rationale behind this belief is that the ice helps reduce inflammation and provides more pain relief. After the initial swelling decreases, applying heat can then help healing by causing more blood flow to the area.

Either of these methods works just fine. Both ice and/or heat can reduce muscle spasms.

Try Anti-Inflammatory Drugs

In addition to bed rest and applying ice and heat, anti-inflammatory medications can help your back pain in the initial stages. Anti-inflammatories include such readily available medicines as aspirin, ibuprofen (Advil, Nuprin, Motrin), and naproxen sodium (Aleve). Any over-the-counter anti-inflammatory medication can help decrease inflammation associated with your back pain, and can provide some pain relief. To avoid side effects, we recommend trying Tylenol first.

Take your medicine according to the directions on the bottle. An important note: If you think your moderate to severe back pain may go on for more than a day, then continue taking the medicine for several doses. Don't stop the medication because you feel slightly better. Taking medication at regular intervals, according to the directions, for about 1 or 2 weeks builds a level of the medication in your blood that can continue to fight inflammation and provide pain relief over the course of your acute back pain flare-up.

On the other hand, do not believe that "if a little medicine is good, then more must be better." Follow the directions on the medication bottle unless your doctor says to do otherwise. Taking more medicine than is recommended can have serious side effects such as liver and kidney damage, among other things.

Many anti-inflammatory medications that are now available over-the-counter were previously prescription drugs. As with all medication, you must take care to follow the directions and read warning information on the label. For instance, one of the most common side effects of anti-inflammatory medications includes stomach upset, abnormal bleeding (especially with aspirin), and ulcers. If you have problems with your stomach or gastrointestinal system, you should check with your doctor before taking any of these medicines. Acetaminophen generally does not have the stomach and gastrointestinal effects that the other medicines can cause. But beware that acetaminophen can cause liver damage at higher doses (more that 4 grams per day, or about 8 tablets that contain 500 milligrams of acetaminophen each).

If your back pain does not improve after taking these medications for 1 or 2 weeks (and following our other recommendations in this chapter), consult your doctor (if you haven't already). If you're on other medications for different medical problems, or if you have a medical problem in addition to your back pain, you should always consult with your physician before self-medicating. Talking with your doctor can help you avoid any serious drug interactions.

Starting to Move and Returning to Normal Activity

After a few days of bed rest, you should start gradually increasing your activity and overall time out of bed. Walking is an excellent exercise that is safe for your back, gets your blood flowing, and stretches out your stiff muscles. Moving around also helps you feel like you're starting to return to a normal life.

You can begin by walking around the inside of the house and progress to walking around the block or farther. Adjust your speed depending on your back pain, starting out very slowly and eventually working your way up to speed walking. Make sure that you begin your walking program on a level surface. When you're in the midst of a back attack, walking up and down hills can aggravate your back pain.

If you have trouble with a walking program initially, consider doing mild exercises in a pool if that option is available to you. This workout may involve simply getting into the pool and walking across the shallow end. This mode of exercising is easier on your body because it is almost weightless in the water. You're placing minimal stress on your back. Also, the water prevents you from doing any jerky or rapid movements.

If your walking is going relatively well, you can add in some simple back exercises. As you start to feel better, you can also begin to engage in more normal activities, usually beginning with doing things around the house.

If you aren't experiencing significant relief or if your back pain isn't improving by now, you need to seek professional help from your physician or a spinal specialist. Your doctor will give you an evaluation and further treatment recommendations.

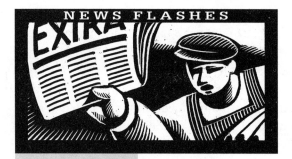

Critical-Care Specialists Increase Odds of Surviving Surgery

BALTIMORE—You need more than a crack surgeon to pull through an operation. Researchers at Johns Hopkins University have determined that critical-care specialists can triple your odds of surviving surgery. Researchers evaluated 2,987 heart-surgery patients and found that those receiving postoperative treatment from physicians certified in critical care had only a 7 percent mortality rate, compared with a 21 percent rate for those treated by regular M.D.'s. "A man who is scheduling any major surgery should ask if critical-care specialists are available. If the answer is no, consider going elsewhere," says Peter Pronovost, M.D., the lead study author.

Skip the Antacid Chaser

STANFORD, Calif.—Nonsteroidal anti-inflammatory drugs (NSAIDs) such as aspirin and ibuprofen can cause ulcers and bleeding. Unfortunately, taking antacids or acid blockers with NSAIDs can actually increase your risk of gastrointestinal problems. According to Gurkirpal Singh, M.D., a rheumatologist at Stanford University, antacids and acid blockers often mask the symptoms of gastrointestinal damage and keep people from seeking medical help. "These people may end up with twice as many serious GI problems," says Dr. Singh. If you're taking NSAIDs and you experience stomach pain, talk with your doctor before taking antacids or acid blockers.

This Lunch May Protect Your Prostate

STANFORD, Calif.—The perfect lunch to prevent prostate cancer: a tuna-fish sandwich on multigrain bread, and a handful of Brazil nuts. These foods are all rich in selenium, and eating more of this mineral may protect your prostate, says Stanford University's James Brooks, M.D. He conducted a 12-year study on 148 men, and found that the 52 men who developed prostate cancer also had the lowest levels of selenium. "The mineral is an essential part of the antioxidant defenses that may prevent cellular damage," he says. It's safe to take a 200-microgram supplement every day.

Ulcer-Kicking Combo May Be Most Effective Treatment

PORTLAND, Ore.—A combination of three drugs may be the most effective way to kill *Helicobacter pylori*, the bacterium that causes ulcers. Oregon Health Sciences University researchers found that combining a proton pump inhibitor (a drug that stops stomach acid production), the antibiotic clarithromycin, and either metronidazole or amoxicillin (both antibiotics) was more effective than the other treatments tested. "If you're not using these triple therapies to treat your ulcer, ask your doctor why," says M. Brian Fennerty, M.D., the study's lead author.

Strong Odors Help Smokers to Stop

PITTSBURGH—Here's one excuse to stop doing your laundry. Researchers have found that sniffing strong odors reduces the urge to smoke. In a University of Pittsburgh study, 58 smokers rated their nicotine cravings on a scale of 0 to 100 before and after they sniffed scents such as coconut, peppermint, and Vicks mentholated rub.

Researchers found that the strongest odors (whether they were pleasant or not) reduced cravings by 20 percent. The part of the brain that controls cravings also happens to be where you process odors, says the study author, Michael Sayette, Ph.D. So if you're trying to quit, put something at your desk that gives off a pungent odor, such as vinegar or some Vicks.

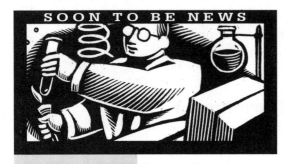

Testosterone to Fight Alzheimer's Disease?

Researchers at Rockefeller University in New York believe that testosterone supplements may eventually help prevent Alzheimer's disease. Their study, published in the *Proceedings of the National Academy of Sciences*, found that extra testosterone added to nerve cells inhibited the process of plaque formation in the brain. "The testosterone appears to limit the ability of the enzymes that form the beta-amyloid protein that creates the plaques," says Paul Greengard, Ph.D., a study author. Previous studies have shown that supplements of estrogen may help prevent the onset of Alzheimer's disease in women.

Researchers have not yet begun testing their findings in animals, and Dr. Greengard says that it may take years before testosterone supplementation is approved for Alzheimer's prevention.

A New Treatment for the Common Cold?

There's still no cure, but there is a promising new medication for the common cold. Ninety-two sick subjects used either a nasal spray called AG7088 or a placebo spray five times a day. After 4 days, those given AG7088 had 30 percent fewer cold symptoms and 40 percent less nasal mucus than the subjects who took the placebos. "It inhibits the enzyme that lets the rhinovirus multiply," says Ronald Turner, M.D., one of the researchers.

Further testing on AG7088 is still needed.

A Urine Test to Detect Cancer?

Advances are being made in the prevention and treatment of cancer. For example, new drugs are being designed to strangle the blood vessels that feed tumors, a process called "angiogenesis inhibition." Clinical trials are being conducted on drugs that use this mechanism to fight melanoma and cancers of the lung, prostate, and kidney. In addition, scientists have developed a test that, for the first time, allows them to monitor urine for chemical indicators of cancer.

Within a few years, screening for some cancers may be as easy as providing your doctor with a urine sample.

Gene Therapy for Male Pattern Baldness?

Researchers at Cornell University in Ithaca, New York, recently found that a new gene-therapy technique may trigger hair growth. Researchers injected a gene that plays a role in the growth cycle of hair follicles into bald patches on mice. Hair sprouted at the site of the injection within 2 weeks; a 6-month follow-up showed no loss. "Male pattern baldness occurs because the follicles have entered their resting phase," explains Ronald Crystal, M.D., the lead study author. "What we've done is turn on the genetic switch that's been shut off."

Human trials may begin this year.

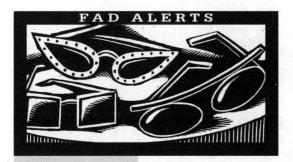

FAD ALERTS

Lycopene

You may have heard that lycopene, the compound that makes tomatoes red, can help prevent prostate cancer. But a recent study at the Karmanos Cancer Institute in Detroit found that it may also treat the disease. Researchers gave 21 men with prostate cancer 15 milligrams of lycopene twice a day (equivalent to the amount in 1½ cups of tomato sauce). After 3 weeks, 17 men had slightly smaller tumors. Lycopene seems to stop prostate cancer cells from multiplying, says study leader Omer Kucuk, M.D. It's a good reason to make tomato sauce, tomato juice, and ketchup staples in your diet.

Glucosamine and Chondroitin

 Compounds that are found in the shells of crabs, lobsters, and shrimp, glucosamine and chondroitin may relieve the pain of osteoarthritis.

Chondroitin inhibits the enzymes that destroy your cartilage in the first place, says David Hungerford, M.D., of Johns Hopkins University in Baltimore. Glucosamine stimulates tissue regrowth in damaged cartilage. When people with osteoarthritis were given 500 milligrams of glucosamine and 400 milligrams of chondroitin twice a day, more than half of them had less pain and more mobility. "I've prescribed them as a first line of treatment for arthritis of the hip and knee for 3 years, and they've been effective," says Dr. Hungerford.

Larger studies are needed, but these supplements do seem to treat arthritis pain safely. If you're diagnosed with arthritis, look for supplements that contain 500 milligrams of glucosamine and 400 milligrams of chondroitin. A 90-tablet bottle of glucosamine will cost about $30.

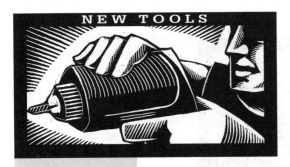

NEW TOOLS

A Way to Correct Color Blindness

Customized Eyeglasses

Men who are color blind—and 1 out of every 12 men is—don't have to see life in black and white anymore. There are now eyeglasses that help correct color blindness. By using a metallic coating that modifies light wavelengths, the lenses enhance the clarity and distinction of muted colors. In clinical trials on 30 patients, the lenses produced significant improvements in all wearers. "The coating is customized to each person's level of color deficiency," explains James Bailey, O.D., Ph.D., of the Southern California College of Optometry in Fullerton. Contact your optometrist for more information.

Prostate Pain Reliever

Quercetin

In a recent study of 47 men at the Institute for Male Urology in Los Angeles, researchers found that 500 milligrams of quercetin—a natural bioflavonoid found in red wine, onions, and green tea—reduced prostate pain in 67 percent of patients suffering from prostatitis. Quercetin is believed to work in part because it increases the endorphins in the prostate fluid, says Daniel A. Shoskes, M.D. He suggests taking quercetin supplements that also contain the antioxidants bromelain and papain, which are believed to further increase absorption of the quercetin.

Nonsurgical Treatment for Osteoarthritis

Synvisc

According to a study presented at the American Academy of Orthopedic Surgeons, a new treatment may help osteoarthritis sufferers avoid knee surgery. Researchers gave 108 knee-replacement candidates Synvisc, an injectable substance that mimics lubricating fluids in the joints. After 18 months, 78 of the patients had avoided surgery. "Patients may now be able to bypass surgery entirely with a simple course of Synvisc treatment," says Edward H. Miller, M.D., the lead investigator. If you have osteoarthritis, ask your doctor about Synvisc.

Reduce Facial Wrinkles without Irritation

Kinerase

Most skin creams that are used to fight wrinkles contain alpha hydroxy acid or isotretinoin, both of which cause burning and peeling. But a new nonprescription cream can reduce facial wrinkles without skin irritation. Eighty-seven people who used furfuryladenine cream (Kinerase) daily for 6 months all showed skin improvements, and only one experienced redness. "It's a good option for men who spend a lot of time outdoors, since it doesn't cause sun sensitivity," says Bruce Katz, M.D., a dermatologist from Columbia University.

A Home Test for Hepatitis C

Home Access Hepatitis C Test

If you received blood before 1992 or you tried IV drugs even once, you should get tested for hepatitis C. About 4 million Americans have the liver-destroying virus, and many of them don't know it. That's because hepatitis C may show no symptoms for years. The Home Access Hepatitis C Test works just like the company's HIV test: You prick your finger, mail your blood sample in the included envelope, and call a toll-free number 10 days later to learn the result. It has a 99 percent accuracy rate, and your health insurance plan may cover the $70 cost. Call (888) 888-4372 to order the test, or call Hepatitis Foundation International at (800) 891-0707 for details about other testing methods.

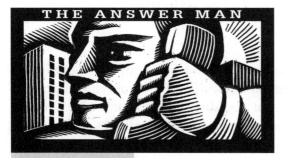

THE ANSWER MAN

Porous Proboscis

I'm self-conscious about the pores on my nose—they seem huge and are always clogged. Is there any way I can clean them and make them less noticeable?

—H. P., Boston

Our advice: Stop looking in the mirror so much. It's true that as you grow older, all of the pores on your body grow larger. But it's unlikely that anyone but you will notice the ones on your honker.

"Patients are always convinced that large, clogged pores are visible to the whole world," says James Leyden, M.D., a dermatologist. "But pores are usually visible only at very close range under very strong light—conditions you're unlikely to encounter outside a dermatologist's office." Or the set of *Larry King Live*.

As for that stuff clogging your pores, it's a harmless mixture of oil and dead skin cells. Dr. Leyden's recommendation for someone who just can't leave his nose alone is a vitamin A cream such as Differin. It might make your pores less noticeable and reduce some of the clogging.

When You Must Operate Heavy Machinery

My allergies are miserable no matter what the season. I've resisted pre-scription drugs so far because I'm afraid of the side effects. Will the hard stuff make me drowsy all day?
—V. A., Greensboro, N.C.

You might assume that prescription antihistamines would cause more grog-giness than over-the-counter allergy medications. You'd be wrong. A study found that 32 allergy sufferers who took Benadryl, an OTC antihistamine, did much worse on concentration and memory tests than 33 people who took the pre-scription drug Claritin. (The study was sponsored, but not run, by the makers of Claritin.) The researchers even compared the Benadryl users' performance to the effects of brain disorders, which gives us a handy excuse for our behavior last weekend. Prescription antihistamines more accurately target the brain receptors that control allergic reactions, says Victoria Starbuck, Ph.D., a neuropsychologist at Georgetown University in Washington, D.C., and one of the study authors. But one drug, Zyrtec, still carries a warning that it may cause drowsiness.

He Screams from Ice Cream

My teeth are so sensitive I feel as if I'm going to pass out when I eat ice cream or anything else cold. Anything I can do to toughen them up?
—J. O., Upper Sandusky, Ohio

Yes. You actually can toughen up your teeth. The reason they're hurting is that your cementum—the protective, calcified coating that covers the roots of your teeth—has been worn down by food acids. That exposes the sensitive dentin underneath and leaves you suffering from screaming-chomper syndrome.

There are two remedies: a fluoridated coating your dentist can apply, or a toothpaste containing potassium nitrate, which you can use at home.

You probably breached the cementum not by eating sweets but by combating them, says Israel Kleinberg, D.D.S., Ph.D., chairman of oral biology at State Uni-versity of New York, Stony Brook. "Diet soda, apple juice, and many mouthwashes—all of these are highly acidic liquids that eventually expose the dentin," says Dr. Kleinberg. "Hard brushing or the scraping dentists do to remove tartar and stains can also corrode the cementum."

You're So Vein

How can I get rid of varicose veins?
—S. T., New Orleans

The most common treatment for varicose veins is sclerotherapy, an office procedure in which the vein is injected with a solution that softens the lining of the blood vessel. Then a special foam is applied to glue the walls of the vein together, basically making it vanish. After the procedure you'll have to wear graduated compression stockings for about a week, which means you'll want to leave your kilt in the closet.

You'll need two to four half-hour sessions, which run about $200 to $300 a pop. Your insurance company may pick up the tab.

Brace Yourself

I couldn't face the humiliation of wearing braces when I was in high school. Now I'm 34 and my teeth are still crooked, but I have even less tolerance for humiliation. What can I do?
—C. B., Wichita, Kans.

A mouthful of metal isn't the only way to straighten teeth, says David Sarver, D.M.D., an orthodontist in Birmingham, Alabama. Here are some less obtrusive alternatives to conventional braces, which normally cost $3,500 to $5,000, plus embarrassment. Most are covered to some degree by dental insurance.

A removable appliance can be worn at night, or full-time if you want your teeth to be straightened more quickly. It's best for moderately crooked teeth, and it costs the same as regular braces. But it's 30 to 50 percent slower, according to Dr. Sarver.

Lingual braces attach to the inner surfaces of the teeth, so they're much less noticeable than the conventional kind. (And they don't make you talk funny.) Because they're more difficult to affix, lingual braces can cost double what you'd pay for conventional braces, and they may have to stay on 30 percent longer.

Regular braces made of tooth-colored ceramic or porcelain won't cost you any more time or money than the metal variety.

Finally, you might want to consider nonorthodontic alignment, which uses porcelain veneers to improve the appearance of your teeth. It can cost from $4,000 to $6,000, says Michael C. Bell, D.D.S., of Austin, Texas. The procedure isn't covered by insurance.

Quit Popping Zits

What's the best way to pop a pimple? I know you're not supposed to touch them, but I can't leave the house with this thing.
—M. C., Portland, Ore.

Squeezing is the worst thing you can do to a pimple, says D'Anne Kleinsmith, M.D., a dermatologist in West Bloomfield, Michigan. "You may squeeze something to the surface, but you'll also end up squeezing the infection deeper into the skin." If you can't keep your hands off, she suggests, hold a warm, wet washcloth to the skin for a few minutes to help bring the pimple to a head. Then, if the pimple appears to be very superficial, you can prick the head with a sterilized needle. Otherwise, just dry the skin and apply a benzoyl-peroxide product.

If the pimple is deep and painful, get thee to a dermatologist, who can inject it with cortisone. This should eliminate the redness and swelling within a few hours.

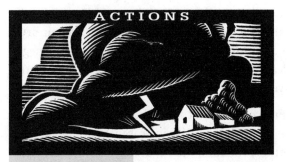

Some days, seemingly minor aches and pains can ruin your whole day. The burning of a cold sore. The lingering—and annoying—symptoms of a cold. A headache that's making you consider volunteering for a lobotomy. It's times like these when a little relief could go a long way. Read on for some simple solutions to these and other day-to-day health nuisances.

1. Think heat for cold relief. Why wait out stubborn cold symptoms when you could burn them out? "Hot, pungent spices help to break up stagnant mucus, enabling you to cough it up," says Irwin Ziment, M.D., chief of medicine at the Olive View–UCLA Medical Center. At the same time, capsaicin—the ingredient that makes hot peppers hot—will help stop sore-throat pain from registering in your brain. Here's Dr. Ziment's recipe for relief: Mix 1 teaspoon of horseradish and 1 teaspoon of Tabasco sauce into a glass of water. Gargle and repeat several times a day until you're feeling better.

2. **Get cultured to defeat diarrhea.** Antibiotics are notorious for causing diarrhea, but according to a study at the University of Pittsburgh Medical Center, eating yogurt can help. In the study, 202 patients on antibiotics added either 16 ounces of yogurt a day to their diets or nothing at all. After a week, 10 percent fewer yogurt eaters had diarrhea, and they spent one-third as many days with the malady. "Yogurt's bacteria preserve the balance of microorganisms that can be disrupted by antibiotics," notes the study author, Ripudaman Beniwal, M.D. Look for yogurt with "live active cultures."

3. **Heal cold sores faster.** One study shows that aspirin may help cold sores heal in half the time. When researchers gave 42 patients with cold sores either 125 milligrams of aspirin daily or no treatment, the aspirin subjects recovered in 5 days compared with 9 for the others. Aspirin may block proteins that fuel the herpes virus. "More research is needed, but if you can tolerate aspirin, it's worth trying," says Stephen Tyring, M.D., Ph.D., professor of microbiology and immunology at the University of Texas Medical School at Galveston.

4. **Dry out swimmer's ear.** After your next dip at the pool, follow this easy routine to prevent swimmer's ear, advises Michael Benninger, M.D., an ear specialist at the Henry Ford Hospital in Detroit. First, dry your ears with a hair dryer set on "low" for a minute or two. Second, concoct a mixture of half white vinegar, half rubbing alcohol. Using a clean eyedropper, carefully put a few drops of this solution in your ear. It will dry your inner ear and prevent any bacterial growth.

5. **Treat pills properly.** First of all, don't store them in your bathroom. Steam from the shower can seep through the medicine cabinet and break down their chemical makeup, essentially making them useless, says Peter Koo, Pharm.D., a pharmacy professor at the University of California in San Francisco. Second, never crush a pill so you can swallow it more easily. Manufacturers cut holes in certain pills with laser beams to precisely release the drug at certain times. "Smash up a pill and it doesn't work," says Bruce R. Canaday, Pharm.D., a pharmacy professor at the University of North Carolina at Wilmington.

6. **Get your fill of folic acid.** Folate—the natural form of folic acid, found in food—depresses an amino acid in your body called homocysteine, says John N. Hathcock, Ph.D., director of nutrition and regulatory science for the Council for Responsible Nutrition in Washington, D.C. The more homocysteine you have in your system, the more likely you are to develop heart disease. So get 400 micrograms (the recommended Daily Value) of folic acid a day. You can get folate from foods such as orange juice and green leafy vegetables. But your body better absorbs folic acid from a multivitamin than it does folate from food, Dr. Hathcock adds.

7. **Instead of counting sheep, just wear socks.** Warming your feet may help you fall asleep faster. Swiss researchers found that 18 men fell asleep quickest when their hands and feet were warmest. This happens because warm feet and hands cause blood vessels to enlarge, allowing more heat to escape your body, which in turn lowers your core temperature faster and causes you to nod off sooner, explains Anna Wirz-Justice, Ph.D., the study author. Putting on socks may help you fall asleep in half the time it normally takes, says Wirz-Justice.

8. **Squeeze your brain.** During a headache, you may feel like grabbing your head and squeezing out the pain. That just might help. Pressing against your skull activates several acupressure points that can alleviate headaches. Place your palms on the sides of your skull, says Michael Reed Gach, Ph.D., founder of the Acupressure Institute in Berkeley, California. Then gently press inward toward the center of your head. Press in gradually for several seconds and breathe deeply, he recommends. Keep doing this all around your skull, especially in areas where you feel the most pain.

9. **Dispel the black-and-blue with some green.** Parsley has a reputation as a remedy for black-and-blue marks, says herbalist Sharleen Andrews-Miller, a faculty member at the National College of Naturopathic Medicine in Portland, Oregon, and associate medicinary director at the college's public clinic. "Just whirl two handfuls of parsley in a blender or food processor with just enough water to make it look like slush," she says. Then pour the mixture in ice cube trays, filling them halfway, and freeze. When you get bruised, wrap the ice cubes in gauze or thin cloth and apply to the bruised spots. Apply them for 10 to 15 minutes, and repeat every 2 to 4 hours, as needed.

10. **Know where to get your fiber.** Unless you've been living in a cave, you know that eating a diet high in fiber will help to prevent constipation. But you don't have to condemn yourself to a life of eating nothing but bran if you want to keep things moving. Check out this list for some non-bran foods that are top-notch sources of fiber.
- Beans: chickpeas, kidney beans, lima beans, black beans, lentils
- Dried fruits: pears, apricots, peaches, figs, prunes
- Fruits: raspberries, blackberries, avocados
- Grains: bulgur, pearled barley, whole wheat spaghetti

11. **To prevent jock itch, start with your head.** That damp towel you dried your feet with can spread the fungus that causes jock itch, warns Tobias Samo, M.D., an infectious disease specialist at Methodist Hospital in Houston. So be sure to dry yourself from head to toe, literally. By drying your feet last, you avoid passing the germs from your toes to your groin. And wash that towel after every use.

12. **Don't blow it.** According to a study from the University of Virginia, it might be best to let a stuffed nose stay stuffed. In fact, blowing your nose could make your cold last longer. Using x-rays, researchers discovered that nose blowing actually forces some mucus backward. "You may propel bacteria and viruses directly into your sinuses, which may trigger reactions that could make your cold worse," says Owen Hendley, M.D., the study author. He suggests limiting your honking and taking antihistamines as soon as symptoms appear.

13. **Look to your arm for stomach relief.** If you're suffering from nausea, a stomachache, or indigestion, two acupressure points on your arm could offer relief, says Michael Reed Gach, Ph.D., founder of the Acupressure Institute in Berkeley, California. The first point is on the underside of your wrist. Bend your hand so that the crease between your hand and your arm appears. In the center of this crease is a small dip formed by your wrist bones. Hold your finger in the center of the crease for a minute or two using firm pressure as you breathe slowly and deeply. The second point is about 2 inches higher than the first. Place your finger directly between the two bones in the underside of your forearm. It should be about three finger widths above the crease of your wrist. Sit comfortably as you press firmly for about 2 minutes.

14. **Get heartburn relief with a vinegar cocktail.** As unpleasant as it sounds, drinking apple cider vinegar aids digestion and eases heartburn by neutralizing excess acid, says Steven Bailey, a naturopathic doctor at the Northwest Naturopathic Clinic in Portland, Oregon, and a member of the American Association of Naturopathic Physicians. "And since the pH in the cider is not the same as antacids', it's more natural and doesn't damage the stomach like antacids can," he says. Mix 1 teaspoon of apple cider vinegar with 8 ounces of water and ½ to 1 teaspoon of honey. Take this once in the morning and once at night, as needed. You can also drink this mixture after a meal if you are having digestive problems.

15. **Go for a garlic footbath.** Raw garlic has natural antifungal properties, so it can help treat a case of athlete's foot. Simply put several crushed garlic cloves in a basin with warm water and a little rubbing alcohol. "This is my first-choice treatment," says James A. Duke, Ph.D., the world's foremost authority on healing herbs and author of *The Green Pharmacy.* "A garlic footbath might be malodorous, but it usually relieves itching and burning between the toes."

16. **Jilt constipation with juice.** Apple juice is a tried-and-true elixir for mild constipation, but it'll work even better when you mix 4 ounces of apple juice with 4 ounces of aloe vera juice, says Maoshing Ni, Ph.D., a doctor of Oriental medicine, licensed acupuncturist, and director of Tao of Wellness, a professional acupuncture corporation in Santa Monica, California. You can purchase aloe vera juice in health food stores. Drink the concoction on an empty stomach first thing in the morning for the quickest relief. In fact, to keep your bowel healthy, make this juice mixture part of your daily regimen. You can drink one glass a day without any side effects, says Dr. Ni.

17. **Cast off corns with castor oil.** Castor oil softens corns, making them less painful and easier to file down. Simply massage your feet with castor oil every night, recommends Andrea D. Sullivan, Ph.D., a doctor of naturopathy; president of Sullivan and Associates Center for Natural Healing in Washington, D.C.; and author of *A Path to Healing*. In addition, the oil and massage can help reduce the tension and pain of bunions as well.

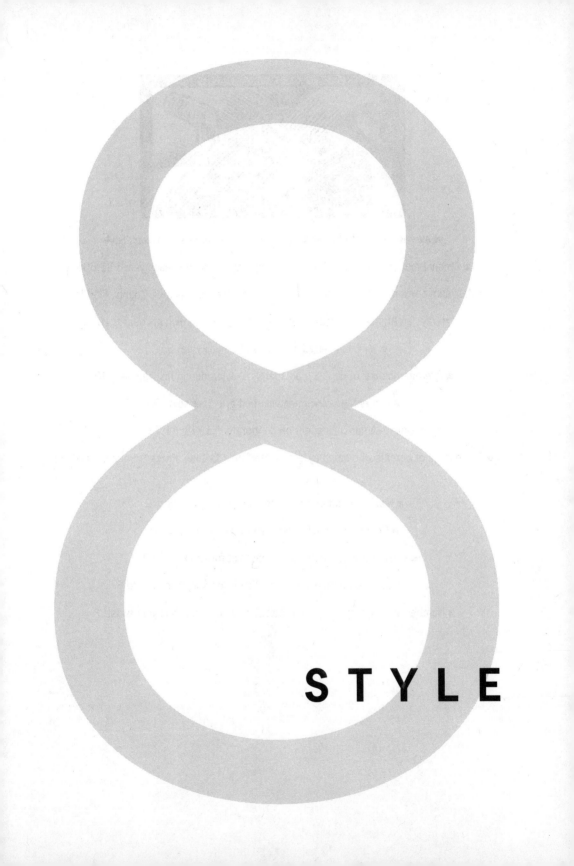

STYLE

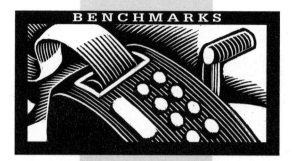

■ Average amount of money men spent on underwear last year: $54

■ Amount that an average U.S. consumer spends on clothes each year : $1,508

■ Maximum portion of buttocks that one may legally bare in Manatee County, Florida: ⅔

■ Days an Afghani man may be held in prison for trimming his beard: 10

■ Minimum length in inches of a quality tie: 55

■ Average number of days a man spends shaving during his lifetime: 140

■ Percentage of women who find gray hair sexy: 90

■ Dollars Americans spent on deodorant in 1998: $1.7 billion

■ Percentage of parents who say they get most of their fashion advice from their children: 13

■ Maximum number of inches for men's pant cuffs: 2

■ Cost of custom-fit porcelain tooth veneers: $700

■ Cost of Botox injections (a treatment for wrinkles): $400

■ Recommended frequency in months of Botox injections: 3 to 6

■ Number of inches by which your belt should be larger than your waist: 2

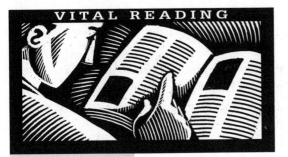

The Lowdown on Skin Care

These products will keep your skin looking great.

Until recently, male skin care was pretty simple. Step 1: Open wrapper of soap purloined from airport Hilton. Step 2: Put some on washcloth and rub vigorously.

You can't get away with that minimalist approach anymore, at least not if you want to age better than a banana. Now you actually have to take care of your hide. There are lots of good health reasons to tend your envelope, and there's one reason that trumps all the health factors: You don't ever want to look like Bob Barker. Not at any age.

Now, if the reason you haven't invested in a few men's skin care products is that you're a mite confused about them all, we can help. Here's the starter skinny on using products to polish up your epidermis, which is, by the way, your largest organ.

Start with Your Skin Type

Before you choose any skin care product, you have to answer the most basic skin question: Do you have dry skin, oily skin, or normal skin? (You may think you already know, but you could be wrong. Skin changes over the years.)

Many products are customized for one type. Oily-skin formulations tend to be light on oils, and dry-skin products are heavier on moisturizing ingredients. Here are two simple tests to find out which formula you should look for, from Dennis Gross, M.D., a dermatologist in New York City. To test for dry skin, wash and dry your face as you normally do. If your skin feels tight and dry immediately after toweling off, you're a dry guy. To detect oily skin, check your face in the late afternoon: Oil or shine on the surface is the giveaway.

If your skin's neither flaky nor slick—and it has no unsightly craters—you probably have normal skin. "Your skin is like your heartbeat: You're basically unaware of it until something is wrong," says Dr. Gross. You should choose products designed for normal skin, although you may need to test a few before you find the best one for you.

For normal guys, Dr. Gross suggests a very basic regimen: Just wash your face, then use a moisturizer. He recommends Basis Soap or Oilatum Soap for washing, and Nivea, Oil of Olay, or Pond's for moisturizing. You can find all of these at your local drugstore.

Soaps and Cleansers

Most men still prefer good old soap to liquid cleansers. If you have oily skin, a nondeodorant soap is fine for washing your face. Try Clinique's Face Soap-Extra Strength (the kind marked for oily skin). Soaps such as Lever 2000 Antibacterial can also be helpful to men with oily skin; because they wipe out bacteria, they may help prevent breakouts. If you prefer a liquid, try one of these treatments for oily skin: Lift Off Power Wash from Lab Series for Men; Neutrogena Oil-Free Acne Wash; Armani for Men; or Escape for Men by Calvin Klein.

If your skin is drier than a convent during Prohibition, look for a nonlipid or nonalkaline soap or cleanser. (Check the ingredients list.) Clinique Face Soap-Regular Strength is designed especially for dry skin. If you want to try a cleanser, consider Cetaphil or Gentle Foaming Face Cleanser from Kiehl's.

Saving Face

Even if your face is not your fortune, you need to protect your chops. Plain old shaving can be a daily assault on your skin, so using the right skin care products can turn that process into a bona fide beauty treatment—or it could, that is, if guys believed in beauty treatments.

Preshave preparations. Preshave treatments are usually oil-based products that hydrate and soften your whiskers and prevent scrapes by creating a thin, protective film. Rub just a couple of drops of preshave treatment into your wet beard right after washing and before you apply shaving cream. The oil holds the moisture, so the blade will glide easily through your whiskers.

Some preshave oils can actually be used in place of shaving cream. If you want to try this, apply the preshave oil to your wet face, work it into your beard, and shave as usual. Use a few more drops of the stuff than you normally would, but be sure to spread it around and massage it completely into your beard, or it can clump up on your razor. Try this technique with the new Close Call Shave

Solution from Lab Series for Men. Close Call Shave Solution can also be used as a traditional preshave, as can both Pre-Shave Aromatherapy from Taylor of Old Bond Street and The Art of Shaving Pre-Shave Oil.

Aftershave products. For more than a century, men have finished their morning shaves by slapping on some aftershave lotion and dancing around the bathroom for a couple of minutes until the stinging stopped. But the post-shave hop is on its way out: An aftershave balm is a much calmer way to start your morning. Like aftershave lotions, aftershave balms usually contain alcohol or witch hazel. But unlike aftershave lotions—which aren't, in fact, lotions—balms are infused with emollients and moisturizers to soothe the skin, not shock it. Feels good, trust us.

If you have oily skin, be wary of balms; they can add oil. Choose one that contains a lot of water. (In general, the higher water is on the ingredients list, the more of it is in there.) Some balms to try: Eternity for Men by Calvin Klein; Drakkar Noir; Lauder Pleasures for Men; Acqua di Giò by Giorgio Armani; Davidoff GoodLife; and Safari for Men by Ralph Lauren.

Around-the-eyes products. You can temporarily reduce puffiness or fine lines around your eyes by applying an eye gel or lotion. These products work in one of three ways: by tightening, smoothing, or exfoliating (stripping away dead skin cells). Gels usually contain alcohol and other ingredients, such as natural sea extracts, to tighten the area around the eyes. Eye creams moisturize the tissues to soften lines. And an AHA (alpha hydroxy acid) eye cream treats fine lines by skimming off the surface layer of skin, leaving a smoother appearance. Gels that treat the eye area include Eye Time Rescue Gel from Lab Series for Men and Ralph Lauren Polo Sport Eye Fitness. H_2O Plus makes a moisturizing cream called Eye Oasis Moisture Replenishing Treatment, and Dermalogica offers an AHA cream called Total Eye Care.

Scrubs. A scrub is a cleanser that contains abrasive particles, such as apricot pieces. Yum. The abrasives help remove old or dead skin cells. Steven A. Victor, M.D., a dermatologist, cautions that being overly forceful with a scrub may cause abrasions. "The power of scrubs is built into them, so you don't have to rub them in like you're buffing your car," says Dr. Victor. Apply a scrub to wet skin, work it over your face in circles, then rinse it off thoroughly. Good scrubs include Face Scrub by Clinique; Active Treatment Scrub from Lab Series for Men; Skin Prep Scrub by Dermalogica; and Cooling Face Scrub from the Black Ice Collection by H_2O Plus.

Face moisturizers. These creams offer sun protection and help maintain the elasticity of your skin. The Technique Pour Homme collection from Chanel includes a moisture formula with alpha and beta hydroxy acids, a sunscreen, and some vitamin A for good measure. Lift Off Moisture Formula from Lab Series for Men offers AHAs, a sunscreen, and vitamin E. If you have oily skin, try Ralph Lauren Polo Sport Face Fitness AHA Moisture Formula. It's oil-free and contains ingredients to soothe your face, plus alpha and beta hydroxy acids and a sunscreen.

Buffing Your Body

Most of us spend so much time checking our faces in the mirror that we overlook the skin on the rest of our bodies. Most skin care products for your body are variations on the formulas for your face. Body scrubs are usually heavier than facial scrubs—meaning that they have bigger, tougher abrasive particles than face scrubs do. Body moisturizers are often lighter, containing less oil and more water than facial moisturizers. This formulation helps speed up the absorption process: You don't want to lose valuable morning minutes standing around waiting for your body moisturizer to dry.

The dry skin/oily skin issue is even more important for body skin care products than for face products. The reason is sweat. If you work out regularly, or if you just sweat a lot, your skin will tend to move toward its end of the dry-oily spectrum. Dry skin will naturally become drier as you sweat. So if you tend toward the dry end, you'll need to replace moisture your skin has lost. Oily skin will produce even more of the slick stuff during a workout, so it will need an especially thorough cleaning afterward.

Cooldown products. If you sweat a lot and have trouble bringing down your body temperature after exercise, you might try one of the new cooldown skin treatments. Jovan's Aftersport Body Cooler is a gel that uses marine extracts to cool down overheated skin. Crunch Care makes Bi-Polar Gel, which uses peppermint oil and aloe vera to stop the sweat. Hilfiger Athletics from Tommy Hilfiger offers Body Cooling Gel with menthol to help cool the skin.

Body scrubs. The larger, more numerous particles in body scrubs have the same purpose as those in face scrubs: removing old, dead cells from the skin and refreshing and rejuvenating it. Good body scrubs include Tommy's Nitty Gritty body scrub from Tommy Hilfiger; Under Your Skin Body Scrub by Biomedic; Safari for Men Oatmeal Soap by Ralph Lauren; and Crushed Seaweed Soap from Phytomer.

One warning: Avoid scrubs if you've just been in the sun. Giving yourself a scrub treatment after you've been sunburned is both painful and dangerous. Try a margarita instead.

All-over moisturizers. Like facial moisturizers, many body moisturizers provide sun protection and help keep your skin looking young. One of the most important differences between young skin and old skin is its moisture content. But if you have oily skin, you may already have all the moisture you want. To get the protection with a minimum of extra oil, Dr. Victor suggests choosing a moisturizer that has a larger percentage of water than of emollient. Check product labels. Corn Huskers Lotion from Warner-Lambert is one good example. If your skin is particularly dry, look for a lotion that has a higher percentage of moisturizer than of water. Two to consider: Kiehl's Crème de Corps, and Moisturizing Body Lotion with Shea Butter from Krismark. If you're one of the lucky few with normal skin, try M Body Lotion from Banana Republic, or Nut Body Butter, a moisturizer from the Body Shop. Just don't tell anyone you shop there.

Body Flaws That Attract Women

Got a bald head and a big gut? You just might be surprised with what women are saying about you.

Forget pretty boys like Brad Pitt. You can hold your balding head and big nose high. Why? Because according to our informal survey, plenty of women find men with so-called body flaws attractive, even downright sexy. Translation: It's time to stop whining about your genetic defects and start flaunting them—particularly if you have one of these seven.

A big nose. Strong features make men look smarter and more intense, and a big nose can fool women into thinking you're big in other important areas. "Testosterone is what makes men have larger noses than women, so a large nose leads to a perception that one is more masculine," says T. Joel Wade, Ph.D., a psychology professor at Bucknell University in Lewisburg, Pennsylvania. Forget Leonardo DiCaprio—few women over the age of 14 prefer pretty men. "Little, perfect noses can make men look feminine," says Olivia, 29. A generous schnozz can even create the appearance of intelligence and thoughtfulness. "It's a nearsighted, intellectual, slightly awkward look that can be very sexy," explains Annie, 30.

A unibrow. Brows that meet in the middle or reach halfway to your scalp have a defiant, Neanderthal quality—intense, slightly primitive, earthy. If you've left them to sprout untamed, either you're confident enough to throw down the tweezers and get on with your life, or you're so unself-conscious that you've never even considered how to part the shrubbery. "A man who isn't obsessed by his appearance may be less egocentric, which appeals to women," says Rita Freedman, Ph.D., a clinical psychologist in Scarsdale, New York.

On a more basic level, a hirsute brow projects the possibility that you're up for passionate caveman sex. "The he-man look of facial hair gives the impression that a man will take charge, and a lot of women like that," says Sandra Reishus, a clinical sexologist and relationship consultant in Sacramento, California.

Of course, the brooding thing will only get you so far. "I dated a handsome Greek artist with a pretty respectable unibrow," says Nicole, 29. "He had strong features, and I actually thought it worked with his face, almost like a frame. I eventually broke up with him, but it wasn't because of the unibrow. It was because he had no sense of humor . . . and he was a bad painter."

A facial scar. A small scar on your chin or cheek might intrigue some women, who will think that you're mysterious or adventurous—even if the scar is only a lasting reminder that you were thrown from the seesaw when you were 4. Heck, you can always lie about it. "A scar sends a message that a man can take care of a woman, that he'll fight battles for her, and that he's not afraid of life," says Reishus. It also might make her think you have a lucrative contract with the NHL. "I dated a hockey player, and the scar on his chin told a story about him," says Shelly, 29. "It was very sexy—I used to run my fingers along it in bed."

A big gut. Sure, many women adore running their hands across rock-hard abs. But according to the women we surveyed, there are some who'd trade in a six-pack for something mellower—say, a bottle of merlot and a guy who'd rather burn off calories on them than on a StairMaster. "A round belly is a sign of someone who enjoys food and the good life—a bon vivant," says Galia, 29. "And I don't feel like I'll have to starve myself to stay skinny for him."

Some women are also drawn to the unmistakable maleness of a gut. "Men are genetically predetermined to get thick in the middle, much more so than women," says Dr. Freedman. "Obvious signals of gender difference can be very attractive to some women." Caution: Don't take this as license to start devouring whole chickens as snacks.

A skinny butt. Some women confessed that lanky guys bring out a nurturing instinct in them. And they also pointed out that they feel they don't need to fear these guys. "She doesn't have to worry about getting crushed when you're on top of her in bed," explains Thomas F. Cash, Ph.D., author of *The Body Image Work Book.*

Another plus: As any guy in a long-term relationship knows, women make a hobby of obsessing about weight. So they might figure that it's easier for them to stay slim if their mates don't have Little Caesar's on speed dial. Being skinny also usually means a guy eats healthfully. "I date a skinny chef," says Janet, 27. "The fact that he's thin but spends 15 hours a day around food makes me more con-scious of what we eat when we're together."

A lack of stature. "In studies where I've asked men and women what they find attractive, there's a tendency to think the opposite sex has extreme standards. Men think that women will say a man has to be 6 feet tall," says Dr. Cash. "That's not true. Women are a lot more accepting of things like lack of height than so-ciety would have us believe."

Dr. Cash also says that small women are often attracted to short guys. "What I love about my boyfriend's height is that we see eye to eye, literally. When we make love, my face is not pressed into his chest. It is right there looking directly at him," says Valerie, 24.

Also, some women feel that short guys tend to compensate for their lack of height in other important ways—socially and sexually. "My first boyfriend after college was maybe 5 feet 5 inches tall, and I fell in love with him the first time I met him because he was really funny and outgoing," says Marie, 30. "And he wasn't 'short' where it counted."

A bald head. A thinning pate at a young age can actually help you draw in women who are looking for mature men. Even if you're still young and idiotic, baldness signifies life experience and maturity. "Women find status attractive," Dr. Wade says. "As men grow older, they're thought of as wiser. A receding hair-line is related to that kind of status evaluation."

"It's true that men with a full head of hair are perceived more favorably by women than balding men on the first impression," says Dr. Cash. "But the dif-ference is very slight. And balding men often start to work out more, dress better, and improve themselves in other ways that more than make up for the differ-ence." They should also shave their remaining hair immediately. "I love the Mr. Clean look," says Annemarie, 28. "It screams confidence."

Clothes Make the Man

So here's what you can do to keep them looking great.

If you think only women, models, and rock stars need to pay attention to their clothes, you've got another think coming. If you want to look your best (and if you want women to hang all over you), you need to take a few minutes a day for routine maintenance of your clothes. Following these directions will save you time, money, and annoying trips to your mom's house to have her reattach your buttons.

Sweaters

Care: Dry-clean sweaters after every fourth wearing. You can hand wash cotton sweaters at home, but they'll fade over time. Lay them flat to air-dry.

Storage: Fold sweaters, whether they're wool, cashmere, cotton, or a blend. Keep wool and cashmere sweaters in a dresser drawer lined with mothballs or cedar chips during the summer. Don't store them in plastic bags. Storing sweaters in plastic actually attracts moths.

How to fold a sweater:

1. Hold the sweater up by each shoulder, with the front facing you. Or lay the sweater flat, front side down, on a flat surface. Fold each sleeve diagonally across the back.
2. From the shoulder, fold the sides of the sweater in toward the back so the points of the shoulders meet in the center.
3. Fold the sweater in half. Now, fill out that application at the Gap.

Leather Jackets

Care: When leather is wet, allow it to dry naturally—don't put it near a heater. For those white salt marks, sponge the area with cool water, then let it dry. Use a leather conditioner if the skins get dry or scratched.

Storage: Hang a leather jacket on a sturdy wooden coat hanger. Never leave it in a plastic dry-cleaner bag—the bag creates a vacuum, and the leather can dry out and crack.

Coats

Care: Wool overcoats need cedar-chip or mothball protection during warm months in storage, and should be dry-cleaned once or twice each winter. If a lining rips, tape or pin it up, then visit a tailor. A dangling lining can cause industrial accidents.

Storage: Overcoats and raincoats should go on sturdy wooden hangers.

Suits

Care: Dry-clean suits once every 3 months, unless you see stains; clean the jacket and pants at the same time. If you don't, they can fade or wear out at different rates. Keep a lint brush or masking tape around in the meantime. And never iron a suit as you would a shirt—it'll look shiny afterward. Buy a steamer, or put a towel between the iron and the suit if you have to get wrinkles out of the pants.

Storage: Hang suits on wooden hangers with wide shoulder supports. Instead of hanging the trousers folded at the knee, which can leave a mark, buy trouser hangers (the small wooden ones that clamp together) or hangers with clips, and suspend pants by the cuffs. Store heavy wool suits for the summer in a closet with an open box of mothballs or cedar chips. And unless you want to smell like an old lady, clean the suits when you remove them from storage.

Shirts

Care: Experts say that it's better to wash your dress shirts at home and press them yourself. Maybe next lifetime. So have your shirts laundered (hold the starch), not dry-cleaned. The cleaner's chemicals can damage the fabric. After washing polo shirts, let them air-dry so they don't fade.

Storage: Ask for most of them on hangers, but keep a few dress shirts in the cleaner's boxes. That way they'll be easy to pack for travel. Since polos are knits, they'll keep their shape better if you store them folded. You can iron them if they get wrinkled.

Khakis, Jeans, and Wool Pants

Care: Wash khakis according to label instructions, but dry them on the cool setting to preserve color and length. To reduce fading, turn jeans inside out before washing them. Dry-clean wool pants once or twice every winter. Cleaning chemicals can fade or weaken wool fibers.

Storage: Khakis and wool pants should be hung the same way as suit pants. Never leave belts in the loops. Fold or hang jeans? Your call.

Shoes

Care: Save your shoes by having your shoe repairman put taps or thin rubber heels on leather soles; use a protective spray on suede or nubuck. If the suede develops bald spots, brush the shoes with an old toothbrush to lift the nap.

How to polish your shoes

1. Rub a quarter-size dab of cream polish onto your shoes with a soft cloth, using a circular motion.
2. Brush the shoes, moving quickly over the leather to give it a sheen.

3. Rub on a light coat of shoe wax, brush again, and wipe with a clean soft cloth.

Storage: Don't wear shoes 2 days in a row. They need to air out. Store in a dry place to avoid mold.

Use wooden shoe trees. Not only do they help leather shoes retain their shape, they also absorb the moisture shoes retain after each wearing. Stuff shoes with newspaper after you get caught in the rain; it'll help suck up the moisture.

Belts

Care: Buff leather with a soft cloth (don't use polish) to keep it supple and scratch-free. Silver buckles should be shined every few months.

Storage: Hang belts from their buckles on hooks. Or coil them and keep them in a drawer.

Ties

Care: Look for an expert tie cleaner; some methods fade the silk, and pressing machines can ruin a tie's shape. Ask your cleaner to spot-treat stains. Or mail your tie to Tiecrafters, masters of tie cleaning and repair in New York City (call 212-629-5800). If you get a water spot, use the thin end of the tie to blot it—the spot should vanish as it dries. When removing a tie, gently work the knot free by reversing the knotting process. Otherwise you'll stretch the tie as you pull the narrow end out of the knot.

Storage: To save space, use wooden tie racks with brass hooks. When traveling, roll your ties to avoid wrinkling.

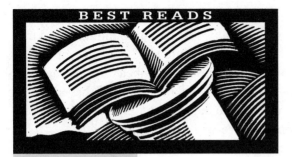

BEST READS

Shoes: A Sign of Your Style

You can skimp on the quality of a suit, as long as it's well-tailored. You can wear cheap underwear because your coworkers and prospective bosses aren't going to see it (we hope). You can even do a great job of finding ties that look good but cost little. But you can't afford to go wrong with shoes. Pick the incorrect ones, and you'll look like a boob no matter what you do above the ankles. In this selection adapted from The Indispensable Guide to Classic Men's Clothing *(Tatra Press), authors Josh Karlen and Christopher Sulavik answer common questions about choosing and caring for shoes.*

Shoes, like the rest of your wardrobe, say a lot about your sense of style. A well-polished pair of cordovan oxfords, for example, signals your attention to detail and appreciation of quality. A battered pair of cheap shoes can tell the world less flattering things.

However, shoes must serve function as well as style. Poorly fitting shoes make life a misery. Even ancient man grasped the tension between footwear's form and function. Some shoes estimated to be as much as 8,000 years old that were found in Calloway County, Missouri, were comfortable-looking slip-ons made of grass, fiber, and leather, yet also had modern design elements, such as heels, a sleekly shaped toe, and straps to allow for a secure fit and easy removal. Even in that age, a man probably would have been pleased to have shoes admired by the less well-shod.

Until the late 19th century, most shoes extended above the ankle to protect the wearer's feet from the elements and from mud in unpaved streets, and those cut below the ankle were worn with spats (ankle coverings attached to the shoe's instep). But by the early 20th century, when urban living became tidier, nearly all dress shoes were cut low and spats were done away with. Through this century, men's shoe designs have changed little.

Q. What are the classic shoe styles?

A. Most shoes fall into two groups: the *oxford*, and the *slip-on*.

Broadly speaking, the *oxford* (named after the British university, where it is said to have originated) embraces all lace-ups that are cut to the ankle and that have at least three lacing eyelets. Oxfords divide into two broad categories, differentiated by the styling of the lace-up area: the *blucher* (open throat lacing), and the sleeker, and therefore dressier, *balmoral* (closed throat, or "V" shaped lacing, named after the British royal family's castle in Scotland). Purists maintain that only the black cap-toe with a balmoral lace-up is a true oxford.

As a rule, lace-up shoes are the summit of dressiness short of formal pumps, and are acceptable businesswear around the world. But lace-ups also can be styled more casually, by use of rougher grain leather, a blucher rather than a balmoral, and other details.

The term *slip-on* covers a gamut of styles but is basically any shoe with no laces and a short vamp (the top part of the shoe extending to the toe). The *penny loafer* is the most popular slip-on, but many other styles exist, from the leather moccasin boat-shoe to fancy ones of crocodile skin, to the now-classic, and always chic, Gucci loafer, with its fine leather and a metal buckle across the upper. Slip-ons, which first became widely worn by college students in the United States in the 1930s, when they are said to have arrived from Norway, are very popular among Europeans, who have created a great many designs over the years, including the woven leather loafer. In Europe, slip-ons are often worn with suits, a combination that is still frowned on by many in the United States, given the slightly more casual nature of the slip-on compared with the oxford. But slip-ons are increasingly worn with suits in the United States. "Slip-ons are so comfortable, yet they're also very dressy," says Margaret Cordone, manager of Belgian Shoes. "It's a matter of personal taste as to whether you can wear a slip-on with a suit," she adds.

Whether you choose an oxford or a slip-on, stay with the classic styles; you'll find that they provide greater versatility than their trendy counterparts, advises Bruno Francois, President of J.M. Weston New York. "A pure classic shoe will definitely put the one who wears it on firm footing," he says. "It can be worn anywhere and is the best start and completion of any outfit; as an analogy, don't women wear a fine, classic piece of jewelry they like just about anywhere?"

Q. I've noticed that a lot of shoes seem to be made in Britain and Italy. Are there differences among British, Italian, and American shoes?

A. Italian-made shoes, in general, are known for narrow, sleek designs and thin soles. In contrast, British and American shoes are, for the most part, heavier-soled and double-soled. They usually have exposed, heavy *welts* (the layer of leather connecting the sole to the rest of the shoe), prominent stitching, longer vamps, and bigger heels than their Italian counterparts. The sturdier design of British and American shoes resulted from the need for protection from cold, wet weather, and their heft complements generously cut British and American suits. Shoes made in Italy reflect that country's more temperate climate and are appropriate for light-weight clothes. There is no difference in quality among these styles; all three countries have fine shoe-making traditions. The superior choice largely depends on what shoe works best with the rest of your wardrobe, and the climate in which you wear it.

Q. How many pairs of shoes—and which styles—belong in a core wardrobe?

A. The shoes that a man should own primarily depends on his profession and on his leisure lifestyle. A chef, for example, may need two pairs of comfortable boots and a pair of sneakers. An executive might need five dressy pairs of oxfords. A man who spends his weekends around the house with his family will probably want a different shoe than a man who spends his weekends at a country club. For most office workers, however, experts say three shoes is the minimum number to own.

John Isaacs, co-owner of Barrie Limited, of New Haven, Connecticut, suggests: "Going from formal on down, the first is the black cap-toe with balmoral lacing in a regular-weight leather and a ¼ inch-thick leather sole. This style can be worn with any traditional suit and even a tuxedo. Second, go with a pair of what I call the country club type of shoe—the traditional, old-money shoe used with a suit or sport coat. This includes the tassel loafer, monk strap or penny loafer in black, brown or cordovan. The third category would be a more casual, everyday brown blucher oxford with a rubber sole. These casuals are best worn with khakis and a blazer, even jeans or corduroys and, in a pinch, you can use them with a suit. A casual of NuBuck (leather treated to create a nap similar to but not as soft as suede) or suede looks great with flannel slacks."

Q. Are custom-made shoes worth the time and expense?

A. The vast majority of men have no need for custom-made shoes. You may want a pair, however, if you require a special fit or if you are among that minority of men who truly appreciate exquisitely crafted footwear—and can afford their stiff expense (into the thousands of dollars for a single pair). A pair of handmade shoes also endures for decades, survives many resolings and, if the style is a classic, will remain elegant.

According to John Lobb, third-generation owner of London custom shoemaker John Lobb Ltd., custom-made shoes benefit both the health of your feet and your sartorial style: "When (a shoe) is entirely handmade and fits properly, it will put a smile on your face," he says.

Q. What makes some shoes dressier than others?

A. For all styles, black is dressier than cordovan and brown, which are dressier than tan and white. "Brown is considered more of a weekend shoe, or country shoe, than a black shoe, which is normally the color of a business shoe, although that's certainly changing in Europe," says Robert Willis, sales manager of Edward Green, a London custom shoemaker. Any other colors, such as blue, should be worn with caution and only with casual clothing. The simpler the shoe, the dressier; the more detail and embellishments (perforations, medallions, tassels, exposed stitching, and so on), the more casual the shoe. "The plain cap-toe is considered more formal than the wing-tip," says Willis. Also, as mentioned earlier, lace-ups are dressier than slip-ons, and balmoral lace-ups are dressier than bluchers.

There is also a hierarchy of leathers. The finest calfskin, kidskin, and cordovan usually are reserved for dressy shoes, the sort worn with business suits and formalwear. Suede and full-grain cowhide are usually used for more casual shoes. Other, more exotic skins, such as those of crocodile and alligator, are expensive, but are generally not appropriate for traditional business.

The following are descriptions of the most common types of shoe leathers:

- Alligator and crocodile: These skins—and other exotic skins such as those of lizards and snakes—are usually very costly. They are often used for slip-ons.
- Calfskin: Calfskin is among the most versatile and common of skins used for shoes, because it is soft and durable and breathes well. It can be given a shiny, matte, or textured finish.
- Cordovan: A heavy, sinewy leather from horse's rump. Shoes of cordovan often are the most expensive and, when well taken care of, can last a lifetime. It has a characteristic mahogany color and glossy shine. The most durable leather available.
- Full-grain leather: Technically, any leather which has not been split (peeled into two layers). However, when you see "full-grain leather" on a label or stamped on the sole, the leather is probably from a cow. Cowhide is considered poor-quality material for uppers because of its toughness. It is usually split, and the result is used for lining or cheaper shoes. Cowhide is often altered by the use of coloring or by pressing textures into it (for example, faux alligator).

• Kidskin: Leather from a young goat, known for its exquisite pliability and breatheability. Kidskin was more popular decades ago, and it is now uncommon in American-made men's shoes, but it is commonly used for custom shoes.
• Suede: Usually inside-out calfskin, which is treated in order to create a soft, chamois-like nap.

Q. Are there any guidelines so that I'll always choose the best shoes to wear with my suits?

A. There are four general rules:
• First, keep your shoes darker than your suit. Light-toned shoes—and socks, for that matter—tend to draw attention to the foot. The shoe should accent the entire ensemble, not dominate it.
• Second, keep your shoes in the same color-family as your suit. So you'd wear black shoes with a navy blue suit or a gray suit, for example, and brown shoes with a brown suit. Some men, however, wear brown shoes with navy or charcoal suits. This is tricky territory. If you venture there, choose a pair of dark brown or cordovan shoes and make sure they are very well polished.
• Third, keep your shoes of roughly the same level of dressiness as your suits—so stay clear of moccasins, be wary of loafers unless your suit has a relaxed cut, and play it safe with oxfords.
• Fourth, keep your shoe style balanced with your suit's silhouette: no tiny Italian slip-ons with your Sack suit.

Q. Is wearing boots with a suit bad form?

A. These days, most men would say yes. However, until almost a century ago, most business shoes were cut above the ankle. The lower-cut oxford became standard business attire only after modern life grew sufficiently tidy. Today, it goes without saying that snow boots are never appropriate indoors when wearing a suit, nor are cowboy boots or most other pointed boots. If you do choose to wear boots with your suit, make sure that the boot style, when partially covered by trouser, exhibits the smooth lines of a dressy oxford. You'll find, especially in the dead of winter, that black, highly polished monk straps or sleek, conventionally shaped boots, with soles of leather (not deep-treaded, rubber lug), will probably not draw disapproving comments or glances.

Q. I walk to work and find leather-soled shoes uncomfortable. Are shoes with rubber soles too casual for business attire?

A. Yes, they are too casual. Traditionally, rubber soles were used for casual or sports shoes, and not for business shoes, and they remain incongruous with a suit. True, more and more men are wearing oxfords and slip-ons with rubber soles, even though these soles are less elegant than leather soles. And rubber soles do have merit: They are quiet and, therefore, good for the self-effacing man; they are not slippery on wet surfaces; and they tend to outwear leather soles. Most important, they cushion shock better than leather. Shoemakers are responding to the increasing acceptance of rubber by combining leather and rubber in the same sole for the best of both types. But leather-soled shoes are generally the proper shoe to wear with a suit.

Q. How can I recognize a well-made pair of shoes?

A. Leather: The quality of the shoe's leather is more important than the craftsmanship put into the shoe. Great leather has a smooth, consistent grain, is luxurious to the touch, and allows even the heaviest shoe to be pliable and resilient. Leathers are graded 1 through 5, with 1 signifying the highest quality, but these grades are not usually marked on shoes.

Remember, it is the quality of the leather, not the type of leather, that dictates the overall quality of a shoe. "First, check the leather closely, because what looks good in the shop window may appear less so close-up," advises Willis.

- Lining: The lining of superior shoes is made of a high-quality calfskin and is cut so that the leather folds smoothly into the seams and edges.
- Stitching: The stitching should hold the shoe together but rarely be noticed, unless it is meant to be seen for design purposes. Stitching in dressy shoes should be inconspicuous; indeed, custom shoemakers almost completely conceal stitching on the top and bottom of the sole. Exposed knots on the inside of the shoe indicate poor craftsmanship and can cause discomfort. Even the stitching of the sole to welt should be recessed in the leather, and there should be no loose threads. The more hand-stitching, the better. Hand stitching is evident by stitches that are not identical. It allows seams to give a little more, making for a longer-lasting shoe. The threads are also less likely to unravel.
- Soles: The soles should be made of leather—they sound authoritative and

tend to make men stand and walk with better posture. They are also more refined than their rubbery cousins. Leather sole thickness varies with styles, and choosing one style over the other depends on your personal preference, the degree of formality of the rest of your outfit, and the climate in which the shoes must survive. The soles of Italian slip-ons, for example, which are about ⅛ inch thick, are thinner than those of wing-tips and bluchers, which are up to ½ inch thick. Soles can be single-, double-, or even triple-layered.

Most good soles are a pale tan hue; this shows that the sole has not been colored to conceal imperfections. It also reveals the craftsmanship of exposed stitching. Soles also should be shaped as closely as possible to the foot, for a more comfortable and elegant shoe. They should be stitched, not glued to the shoe.

The best heels are made of leather. Many are reinforced with rubber and/or metal tips. Oversized heels can make a shoe uncomfortable and alter the balance of the shoe. Some heels are even attached to the sole with small brass tacks for added durability.

Q. What should I know when I'm trying on shoes to make sure they're right for me?

A. A man can wear a pair of shoes that fit him perfectly, but if he is constantly uncertain and self-conscious about them, then that demeanor—a more unsightly display than any unsightly shoe—will show through. So it's crucial that you feel confident that the shoe style reflects your personality, and that it will be a style appropriate for where you will wear it. After you settle on the appropriate style, consider the following:

- Wear socks of the same thickness as those you will usually wear with the shoe.
- Try on shoes later in the day, after your feet expand.
- Shoes of thinner, suppler leather, such as slip-ons, stretch more than heavily built shoes, so make sure you account for this by choosing a snugly fitting shoe rather than a loosely fitting one.
- Don't let a salesperson convince you that a little breaking in, stretching or shoe cream will transform a painful shoe into a comfortable one.
- Well-fitting shoes should have creases, or break lines, straight across the top of the foot.
- If shoes feel uncomfortable even after you've tried them on in a number of different sizes, don't buy them.

Q. How should I care for my shoes?

A. Well-made shoes will last decades if cared for properly. Consider the advice below to best prolong the life of your shoes:

- Let them rest. Don't wear the same shoes on consecutive days. Perspiration, absorbed into the leather when shoes are worn, needs time to air. Letting the shoe breathe for at least a day will prevent a slow rot from the inside out, and will also prevent them from smelling bad.

- Use shoe trees. It is crucial that shoes are stored fitted with shoe trees, preferably of cedar, which will absorb moisture, and impart a pleasant fragrance in addition to preserving the shape of the shoe. If you don't have shoe trees, stuff crumpled newspaper into your shoes.

- Use shoe horns. Use a shoe horn when putting on your shoes to prevent wearing away, or buckling, the back of the shoe.

- Brush, clean, and polish. Brush off dirt after you wear your shoes and, when needed, clean them with shoe cream. "Polish them regularly with a cloth," advises Willis. The cracking you might find on poorly cared for shoes is caused more from perspiration not properly dried off, than from exposure to the elements. Give them a shine with wax polish about once every three wearings. Shines do great things to leather over the years; as with an old baseball glove, the leather begins to take on a rich patina. A shine protects the leather from moisture and sun damage and retards scuffs. Some shoemakers recommend a hard, wax-based polish; others prefer the softer, fragrant bee's wax polish. Polish your shoes by first wiping them clean with a soft cloth. Then rub in polish, wax, or cream with a slightly damp cloth. Wipe off the excess, let it dry, and buff with a soft-bristled brush.

- Dry your shoes. If you get caught in the rain, don't put your shoes near a heat source. Wipe them dry and leave them at room temperature. After a few hours, insert shoe trees to help keep their shape. Don't polish your shoes when they're wet.

- Rejuvenate suede. The nap of suede shoes can be renewed by softly brushing the shoes with a fine-bristled brush, or by softly rubbing them with a fine nail file.

- Remove salt stains. Salt, used to melt ice and snow on walkways, can leave unsightly white stains on shoes. Even worse, salt can do serious damage because it leeches out moisture from the leather, leaving it brittle and likely to crack. To remove salt residue (which is not visable until it sets in), first dry the shoes. If the shoes are very wet, wipe them with a dry cloth and stuff them with crumpled newspaper; if they are only slightly damp, insert shoe trees. Either way, let the shoes air out at room temperature for about an hour.

Afterward, gently rub the outside of the shoes—especially near the soles, an area where salt is most likely to lodge, and which gets the most wear-and-tear—with a cloth dampened with fresh water. This should remove most of the salt. Then, work into the leather a liberal amount of shoe cream or shoe wax. After about an hour, wipe away the excess; this should remove the remaining salt from the leather. Finally, polish the shoes as you normally do.

Tame Unruly Hair

If you roll out of bed on a Saturday morning and your hair looks like you're a contestant in a Don King Look-Alike contest, you can always hide it under a baseball cap. But what do you do when it's a work day? In this selection from The Doctors Book of Home Remedies for Men *(Rodale), editor Jack Croft offers a number of easy tips to get your hair under control.*

Maybe your cowlick has suddenly headed off for greener pastures. Or your bike helmet has left you looking like Bill Murray is your stylist. Or your hair is just generally contrary and resists staying in place more than a dog in a tub. Don't pull your hair out by the roots; there's help.

Most things about your hair—how much you have, its color, thickness, and character—are hereditary. If you have a shock of coarse blond thatch, chances are that one of your parents gave it to you. But some of the things men do to their hair make it even more unmanageable, says David H. Kingsley, a certified trichologist (a specialist in hair and scalp) and owner of British Science Corporation, which counsels and treats people with hair and scalp problems, on Staten Island, New York. Hair dyes, chlorine-laden pools, harsh sunlight, poor nutrition, and even improper shampooing can add to a litany of hair woes.

Sure, having unruly hair isn't very serious, medically speaking. Aside from mussing up your pride, it's rarely a sign of a deep-rooted medical problem when it begins in adulthood and involves the whole scalp, says Susan P. Detwiler, M.D., a dermatologist in private practice in San Diego. One exception: "If there has been an acute change in the character of the hair, I would suggest getting a thyroid test," she says. So if your hair suddenly becomes excessively coarse or dry, especially if it's coupled with hot or cold spells, lethargy, or irritability, Dr. Detwiler recommends that you see a doctor.

Bring Some Discipline to Unruly Hair

Here are some simple things you can do to remind your hair who's boss.

Go wrong. Going the opposite way with your hair can help get it going back in the right direction. Dr. Detwiler suggests the following technique: Wet a comb. Run it through your hair in the opposite direction of the way you style it. Do that a few times and then retrain the hair back in the normal direction.

Gel it. Find a misting bottle like the ones used to spray plants. Fill it with clean water. "Then spray your hair with a little water, put some gel on it, and run a comb through it," recommends Fredric S. Brandt, M.D., clinical associate professor of dermatology at the University of Miami School of Medicine.

While most gels will help keep your hair in place, finding the one that gives you the look you want may require trial and error, says Kingsley. Read the label for a clue, he suggests. If it promises the wet, slicked-back look that works for you, give it a try. No matter which type of gel you choose, Kingsley recommends starting with less than the package instructs.

Cut it short. Unlike Nero, some men don't want to fiddle around too much. Stephen Moody, assistant general manager of the Vidal Sassoon Academy in Santa Monica, California, says that if that's the case, a short haircut is often easier to style and care for.

Undo the damage. Damaged hair makes for unruly hair. You can avoid that damage, says Dr. Detwiler, by taking a few precautions. Wear a wide-brimmed hat in the sun. Use hair dyes judiciously or not at all. Ditto for hair straighteners and perms.

Spray away. A little hairspray may help tame that mane. Don't overdo it, though. Kingsley recommends that you start with just a touch and work up from there.

Prevent Bad Hair Before It Starts

You might be able to get away with wearing a cap on a bad hair day. But if you follow these tips, you might never have to get to that point.

Become a beachcomber. Heck, you can even try this one at home. Brush your hair. Later, when your hair is messy again, comb it. You'll find the comb catching and snagging more than the brush. For this reason, says Kingsley, people comb much more carefully than they brush. The daily rigors of rough brushing can lead to hair breakage and damage, making your hair even more unmanageable. So brush gently when you want to style your hair, but always comb first. Kingsley suggests using only a wide-tooth, good-quality comb, making sure that the teeth don't have sharp edges from the mold used to make it. He prefers a rubber comb. Metal combs can add static to your hair, making it fly off all over the place. Keep a small comb in your wallet for quick touch-ups in the men's room, recommends Kingsley.

Air it out. Dr. Detwiler was part of a group that studied the damage that can be caused by blow-dryers. She found that home dryers can generate heats of up to 300°F. The problem arises when you allow hair and other bathroom crud to build up on the air intake of your dryer.

Insufficient air flow jacks the internal temperature of the dryer through the roof. The resulting superhot air can damage your hair by forming bubbles in the individual shafts. Not only are those hairs going to be impervious to styling, they often break off at the level of the bubble. The solution is to keep your dryer clean and watch for signs of overheating, such as red coils or a burning smell.

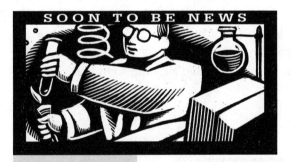

SOON TO BE NEWS

A Gene Fix for Gray Hair?

Researchers at Jefferson Medical College in Philadelphia have used a synthesized nucleic acid to restore hair pigmentation to albino mice. Applied topically and injected into the mice, the acid repaired the gene mutations that caused the white hair. Eventually, the same gene-fixing method may be able to restore gray hair to its original color, according to the study, which was published in *Nature Biotechnology.*

In the future, this technology could also be used to help treat serious skin diseases, liver diseases, and other problems caused by gene mutation, according to Kyonggeun Yoon, Ph.D.

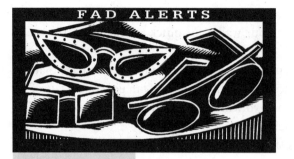

Dryel

When most guys spill something on their clothes, they drown the stain with club soda and end up with an even bigger mess. That's because they're too lazy to go to the dry cleaner. But now there's Dryel, a fabric-care kit for dry-clean-only clothes that's sold in drugstores and supermarkets.

The instructions are simple enough: First you apply the kit's stain-removal fluid to the stain. We tried it on ink, red wine, and a mystery stain on a cotton shirt. Eventually, the Dryel fluid got rid of the ink stain and the splash of wine, but the mystery blotch (if memory serves, a chunk of hamburger fell on the shirt) remained.

So we took the next step: placing the shirt and a Dryel "odor-lifting" cloth into one of the Dryel bags and tossing the bag into the dryer for 30 minutes. The outcome: The stains were gone, but the shirt had a strong scent that was reminiscent of carpet cleaner.

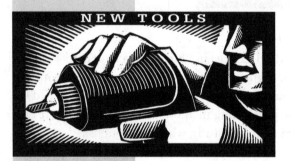

Instant Wallet-Size Photos

Polaroid PopShots

The Polaroid PopShots seems like the perfect camera for a bachelor party: It's disposable and offers impressive blackmail opportunities. Otherwise, who needs a bulky, one-use camera that spits out 10 wallet-size photos? If you're raising your hand, you can find PopShots in drugstores for $20 (each camera comes with a $4 mail-in rebate). The cameras are recyclable; if you return the used camera to Polaroid in the enclosed postage-paid envelope, you'll receive a coupon for $2 off your next PopShots camera. See www.polaroid.com to find a local retailer.

Sunless Tanner

Banana Boat Sunless Tanning Mousse

A tan makes you look healthy, but skin cancer is a nasty downside. To avoid paying that price, use a sunless tanner. These contain dihydroxyacetone, a chemical that temporarily and safely darkens your skin. Our editor tested several and liked Banana Boat Sunless Tanning Mousse best. The "soft-medium" version gave our man natural results that appeared in 3 hours and lasted 5 days. It's not greasy, so it won't give you the uneven coloring that other sunless tanners will. You'll still need sunblock: This sunless tanner offers no UV protection. $6 for 3.75 ounces; call (800) 723-3786.

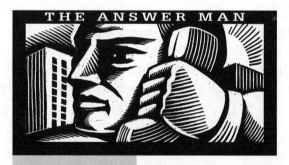

Don't Sweat It

I shower twice a day and I wear enough deodorant to cover the Statue of Liberty. So why do I still pit out my T-shirts with those yellow stains?
—C. K., Morgantown, W.Va.

"You probably have a reaction to a chemical in the deodorant you use," says John F. Romano, M.D., *Men's Health*'s dermatology advisor. "When you sweat, this reaction creates that yellow stuff. The more deodorant you have on, the bigger the yellow stain is going to be." The fix is simple: Change deodorants. Dr.

Romano suggests that if you're currently getting stained by a stick deodorant, try a roll-on or a spray. Try switching brands, too.

"You can also experience staining if you have a problem with bacterial overgrowth, but that's normally accompanied by a smell," says Dr. Romano. "If that's the case, ditch your deodorant and scrub with antiseptic soap for a while. Deodorant is nothing more than an antiseptic designed to kill surface bacteria."

A Nude Noggin

After years of worrying about my thinning hair, I've decided to shave my head. How often will I have to shave it? Will it chafe my noggin?
—L. P., Pierre, S.D.

Depends on what you mean by "shave." If you're not sure how close to the skull you want to go, start by trimming your hair with electric clippers. Do it when your hair is dry, using the widest protective attachment and working your way down to the slimmest attachment—or no attachment at all, which yields the five-o'clock shadow look a lot of men prefer. (You can buy electric clippers at any discount store.) Buzz from the back of the head to the front, says Adam Kaufman of Adam Kaufman Hair Studio in Philadelphia. Use the clippers every 10 days or so to avoid the Chia Pet look.

The next step is the full cue-ball look, which you achieve by shaving your head with the same razor and shaving cream or gel you use on your face. Shave in the direction your hair grows. Hair on the back of the head grows downward, so shave that way in the back. On the top of your head, shave toward the back and to the sides. After you dry your head off, apply a little moisturizer to replace the natural oils you scooped up with the hair. To maintain your chrome dome, shave every day with an electric razor. Buffing with a chamois cloth is optional.

Hat How-To's

How can I clean my favorite baseball cap? It's wool, and I'm afraid it will shrink if I wash it.
—G. T., Baton Rouge, La.

If the hat is stained with something other than sweat, you'll want to be gentle. The key word, according to Judith Pinder of the Woolmark Company, is "dab." First, lightly scratch at the stain with a finger. This works for thicker stains, such as tomato sauce. Then dab at the stain with a lint-free cloth (not a paper towel) dipped in soapy water. For thinner stains, such as coffee or beer, dab with a cloth that's just wet. Soak an ink stain in rubbing alcohol, or spray on some aerosol hairspray, and then dab at it. If the cap is dirty all over and smells bad from your sweaty head, find a dry cleaner who does caps. If you just want to get rid of the smell, toss the hat in the dryer (on a low setting) with a fabric-softener sheet.

Inside the Beltway

How wide should a dress belt be? And what's the style?

—M. F., Concord, N.H.

We checked with Andy Stinson of Torino Belts, who told us that for dress or dress casual (anything but jeans), you should pick up a belt that's 1¼ inches wide. You can wear a wider one with jeans if you like. As far as style is concerned, Stinson suggests narrower belts with unstitched edges and no braiding. Buckles should be rounded and on the small side. Nowadays they lean toward silver rather than gold or brass. Belts with metal tips or metal keepers (a keeper is the little thing you slide the end of the belt under after you buckle it) are not as popular as they were a few years ago, but they're still fine for golf and other casual looks.

A Cuff Conundrum

What is the proper width for pant cuffs? Does it have anything to do with how tall I am?

—J. B., Minneapolis

Anything between 1½ and 2 inches is acceptable, says Tom Mastronardi of Beauchamp, Mastronardi, and Associates, a fashion-industry consulting firm. The exact measurement is a matter of personal taste, but do consider the width of the trouser leg itself and the weight of the fabric. In general, a wider leg needs a wider cuff, and so does a lighter fabric. A wide cuff helps lightweight pants hang better. If you're not sure, ask a good tailor or a knowledgeable salesperson. As far as your height is concerned, if you play in the NBA, wider cuffs will help balance the lower and upper halves of your body. If you're 5'10" or shorter, consider a narrower cuff.

Happy Feet

I have two pairs of dress shoes: black and brown. My dad always told me to wear black shoes with black or gray suits, and brown shoes with blue or beige suits. But these days I see guys wearing all sorts of combinations. What are the modern rules for shoe and suit color combinations?

—K. R., Washington, D.C.

Your father's conservative approach will certainly prevent you from making any huge style gaffes, but you'll find plenty of company if you sport black loafers with your khakis or even brown cap toes with a gray suit. "The modern rule is that there are no rules," says Dennis Sak, a vice president at Salvatore Ferragamo. "The trendier the suit, the more freedom you have to play around with the shoes. It mostly depends on your personal style."

Don't Do It His Way

I've seen some old photos of Frank Sinatra wearing a tie clip, and he looks kind of cool. I have a bunch of tie clips my dad left me. Can I pull off the Rat Pack look?
—D. M., Gary, Ind.

First off, Frank didn't look cool; he was cool. There's a difference. And just for the record, there are three types of tie holders: bars, clips, and tacks. A tie bar extends across three-quarters of the tie's width at midchest. A tie clip is about half the size of a tie bar, and it clips to your shirt. A tie tack has a sharp pin that sticks through your tie and shirt. All were designed to keep your tie out of the marinara sauce—or, in Sinatra's case, out of Ava Gardner's cleavage. Should you wear one? "They're unnecessary and pretentious," says Warren Christopher, *Men's Health* style editor. "My advice: Don't eat spaghetti while wearing a tie; avoid fistfights; and avoid tie paraphernalia at all costs."

Killer Wales

Are corduroy pants still in style? If so, should I wear the thin- or the wide-wale style?
—A.S., Redmond, Wash.

"Corduroys are great fall and winter pants," says Richard Bowes, vice president and fashion director of Bergdorf Goodman Men's Store. Cords have had something of a resurgence over the past few years, especially the thin-wale style (skinny ridges, like the Levi's you wore in the late 1970s). Trousers of wide-wale corduroy are often pleated and cuffed, while pants of the finer-ridged fabric look cool in the flat-front (unpleated) style. Whichever style you choose, Bowes advises that you wear cords as you would wear khakis—with a wool turtleneck and low boots on weekends or paired with a sport coat and knit tie for casual workdays.

A lot of men mistakenly steer clear of wide wales, fearing that the fabric will make them look wider, too. "Wide-wale corduroys don't make you look heavier, as long as they're tailored well," Bowes says.

Finally, whether you buy all-cotton or a wool-cotton blend, corduroy pants should be dry cleaned.

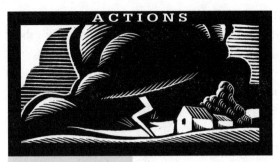

A stylish man knows what clothes make him look his best. He knows that grooming isn't just for horses. He knows that having style means carrying himself in a certain manner no matter what the circumstances. It's about not being taken for a ride, whether he's buying an airline ticket or a car. Here are some pointers on how you can develop that elusive, yet essential, quality.

1. **Become a savvy car shopper.** Everyone knows the typical advice about car shopping at month's end, when dealers are trying to make their sales quotas, and having a mechanic check out a used car before you buy it. But what advice do former dealership pros give their own families? First off, use the Internet to your advantage. Check out Web sites such as www.carpoint.com and www.intellichoice.com to find out what the dealer paid for the car, or the invoice price. Then negotiate up from that price, never down from the sticker. Offer 1 percent over invoice first. If the salesman won't bite, go up to 3 percent over invoice as a final offer. And while you're haggling, don't fall for all those additional fees. Refuse to pay preparation charges or a dealer-exchange fee, the ADM (Additional Dealer Markup, another name for profit), or for Scotchgard or rustproofing (cars are usually rustproofed at the factory), says Leslie Sachs, author of *How to Buy Your New Car for a Rock Bottom Price*. It they won't subtract these, walk.

2. **If you're the boss, take the heat.** Okay, maybe the presentation on market share bombed. But a good boss never lets the higher-ups know that his underling Frank goofed on the visuals big-time. You can deliver as much heat to your staff as you want, after you've taken it like a man from the guy above you.

3. **For the best fit, help out your tailor.** A tailor is the one man who can help you fool the world into thinking you're taller, smarter, and better looking than you actually are. So help out the guy with the following tips from Chris Pamboukas, manager of Nordstrom's tailor shops.

• "When you have a suit tailored, wear a dress shirt and tie, a belt or braces, and dress shoes with the correct height heel. You'd be surprised how many men show up for fittings in cowboy boots or running shoes," says Pamboukas.

• When buying a suit, make sure the collar hugs your neck, the lapels lie flat on your chest, and the armholes allow enough room for movement. A jacket can be tailored to a perfect fit if these three areas fit properly from the beginning.

• Don't buy pants several inches too large in the waist, even if your tailor thinks he can cut to fit. Pants more than 6 inches too large involve a recut, which means removing the waistband and zipper and recutting the fabric. And that's detailed work that can get expensive and requires a highly skilled tailor.

• If you've gained weight, you can let out pants up to 2 inches in the waist, and a jacket can be restructured to give you another 1¼ inches around the middle. You can take the pants in once you lose weight, but the odds of that happening for most guys are pretty slim.

4. **Pour the best brew.** Impress your friends and family—okay, maybe just your friends—with your knowledge of the fine art of pouring a beer. By pouring beer into the center of a glass, you get more bubbles, which release the aroma and enhance the taste. But this may put too much head on the beer. So, for optimum pouring, begin by letting the beer flow down the side of the glass. Then move the stream into the center so you end up topping off the beer with a half-inch head.

5. **Be a polished public speaker.** If you're the guy at the podium, keep your hands out of your pockets, where they might be tempted to rattle keys or coins. And don't cross your arms or put your hands on your hips unless you're emphasizing a point. "Being more aware of where your feet are and what you're doing with your arms and hands is key," says Marjorie Brody, a certified speaking professional and president of Brody Communications, a business and communications skills training company.

6. **Shed your beard the right way.** If you've decided it's time to end the Grizzly Adams look, first read the steps below. They'll help you lose your beard with the least amount of fuss.

• Wet your face, then apply a softening product or a conditioning shampoo to your beard, which will make it easier to cut. Pat dry with a towel.

• Pull the hair straight with a comb and cut an inch at a time with sharp barber scissors or an electric razor. (You can pick up barber scissors for about $10 in drugstores.)

• As you cut closer, slide a comb between your skin and the scissors; cut the hair that peeks through the comb. Work down from your cheekbones.

• When you're down to stubble, wet your face with hot water and apply a thick shaving cream. Shave off the whiskers, going with the grain.

• Apply a moisturizing cream that contains aloe to soothe your skin. Since your beard has been protecting your skin until now, be sure to wear sunscreen for a few weeks.

7. **Schedule the right time for an interview.** Don't rush to be the first guy interviewed for a job. The last interviewee gets the job nearly 56 percent of the time. The worst times for job interviews are Mondays and just before quitting time.

8. **Be sweater smart.** Is that wool sweater the saleswoman is trying to push on you really going to hold up after a few spins in the washing machine? There are a few ways you can tell if you're getting your money's worth. First, look for a piece of fabric at the neck opening called the neck trim. There are two ways that it can be attached: looped with the same yarn that the sweater is made from or sewn by machine. Looping is better. If it's machine-attached, it will come apart in laundering, says Patrice Auerbach, vice president of sales for Tricots St. Raphael in New York City. Next, turn the sweater inside out and look at the seam along the arm hole. Try to put your finger through where the arm attaches to the body. If it's loose, the sweater is poor quality. Finally, check the cuffs of the sleeves and the bottom of the sweater. Good sweaters will have a thin band of elastic in each of these places.

9. **Outsmart the airlines.** So what if there's no T.G.I. Friday's? Obscure little airports sometimes offer less-expensive flights than big ones. For example, a recent trip to Portland, Oregon, cost $400 from New York's JFK International Airport, but only $200 from the tiny airport in Islip, which is only 45 miles away. A travel Web site, www.1travel.com, offers a searchable database of small airports and the fares they're currently offering. The site also lists low-cost fares offered by small regional airlines, such as Vanguard, Frontier, and Eastwind.

10. **Give yourself a (well-manicured) hand.** It's true that women check out men's hands. But not for the reason you're thinking of. They're hoping to find any sign that he has tried to look presentable. Here's how to pass the test in 10 minutes flat. First, shape your nails with an emery board. You should be going for a shape that's rectangular but slightly rounded at the corners. It's easier to control the length of your nails by filing than by using a clipper. File in one direction only—back and forth can leave a rough edge. Next, rub some vitamin-E oil or hand cream on your cuticles—the skin that surrounds the nail itself.

Then soak your hands in a bowl of warm water and liquid hand soap for a few minutes.

Your next step is to clean underneath your nails with an old toothbrush. Take an orange stick (a skinnier version of a Popsicle stick, available at drugstores), wrap cotton around it, and gently push back each cuticle so it's not stretched over the nail. If you have any hangnails, trim them off carefully with nail or cuticle scissors. Finally, wash your hands and rub on a cream that contains mineral oil and vitamins A, D, and E.

11. **Scarf it up.** Wearing a scarf can add a little flair to your overcoat during the winter months. But make sure you pick the right one. Your scarf should always complement your overcoat, notes G. Bruce Boyer, a fashion consultant and author of the book *Eminently Suitable*. The key here is "complement," not "coordinate with." You don't need to pick a perfect color match to your coat. Check and plaid scarves work well with almost any neutral, solid topcoat. Just don't wear a patterned scarf with a patterned coat. Finally, wear your scarf in a simple, straightforward style. Just cross it over the front of your neck, and let both ends hang down the front, inside your coat. "The simplest way is the best," Boyer says. "It's appropriate and it always looks good."

12. **Iron out the wrinkles.** Most men take their shirts to the cleaners not because the shirts are dirty, but because they couldn't iron a shirt to save their lives. But ironing is a simple skill to learn. First off, remember these tips: When ironing cotton dress shirts, use the hottest setting and plenty of steam. Iron lengthwise, not in circles. A little spray starch makes the job easier. Now grab your iron and follow this step-by-step guide.

• Start with the underside of the collar. Iron from the collar points toward the back of the neck. That way any pleats or folds will be hidden at the back of the collar. Now turn the shirt over and iron the front of the collar the same way.

• Next, iron the yoke (the piece that goes across each shoulder and the top of the back). Start from the top of the shoulders and head to the center of the back.

• Press the cuffs, doing the inside first, then the outside. Lay the sleeves flat, then press the body of each sleeve, starting with the cuff-opening side. Then iron the reverse side.

• Finish with the body of the shirt, starting with the back and heading south from the shoulders. Flip it and iron the right front panel, going under and around the buttons with the tip of the iron. (Some irons even have special indentations at the tip for ironing around buttons.) Finally, iron the left front panel and button placket.

13. **Pay attention to the details.** Very little changes in men's fashions from year to year, so the way to distinguish yourself is to pay attention to the details. For example, think about color. Most guys will wear a tan shirt. Distinguish yourself by wearing a unique coffee or mocha color. (They have the added advantage of covering coffee and mocha drink stains much better.) Reach for unexpected juxtapositions and unpredictable color matches, like that mocha shirt with a burgundy tie. "While nothing seems to go together, it all goes together," says Murray Pearlstein, owner of Louis, Boston, an upscale men's and women's clothier. "People will stop and look and comment on your attractive appearance, but they won't know exactly why."

Credits

"Stick-to-Your-Ribs Sides" on page 66 is excerpted from *A Guy's Guide to Great Eating: Big-Flavored, Fat-Reduced Recipes for Men Who Love to Eat* by Don Mauer. © 1999 by Don Mauer and Associates, Inc. Reprinted by permission of Houghton Mifflin Company. All rights reserved.

"Fat City" on page 130 is excerpted from *Choose to Lose Weight-Loss Plan for Men* by Ron and Nancy Goor. © 2000 by Ronald S. Goor and Nancy M. Goor. Reprinted by permission of Houghton Mifflin Company. All rights reserved.

"Memory Loss: Should You Worry?" on page 166 is reprinted from *Staying on Top of Your Game* by Timothy Gower. © 1999 by Avon Books. Reprinted by permission of Hearst Communications, Inc.

"The Fear of Growing Older" on page 169 is excerpted from *Dr. D's Handbook for Men over 40: A Guide to Health, Fitness, Living, and Loving in the Prime of Your Life.* © 1998 by Peter Dorsen, M.D. Adapted by permission of John Wiley and Sons, Inc.

"Three Herbs for a Healthy Prostate" on page 229 is excerpted from *Natural Prostate Healers* by Mike Fillon. © 1999. Reprinted with permission of Prentice Hall Direct.

"First-Aid for Your Back Attack" on page 235 is excerpted from *Back Pain Remedies for Dummies* by Michael S. Sinel, M.D., and William W. Deardorff, Ph.D. © 1999 by IDG Books Worldwide, Inc. All rights reserved. Reprinted here by permission of the publisher. For Dummies is a registered trademark of IDG Books Worldwide, Inc.

"Shoes: A Sign of Your Style" on page 269 is excerpted from *The Indispensable Guide to Classic Men's Clothing.* © 1999 by Josh Karlen and Christopher C. Sulavik. Reprinted with permission of Tatra Press. All rights reserved.

Index

Boldface references indicate photographs. *Italic* page references indicate tables.